W9-BXX-169

CULTURE AND ATTACHMENT

CULTURE AND HUMAN DEVELOPMENT
A Guilford Series

Sara Harkness
Charles M. Super
Editors

CULTURE AND ATTACHMENT:
PERCEPTIONS OF THE CHILD IN CONTEXT
Robin L. Harwood, Joan G. Miller, and Nydia Lucca Irizarry

SIBLINGS IN SOUTH ASIA:
BROTHERS AND SISTERS IN CULTURAL CONTEXT
Charles W. Nuckolls, *Editor*

Forthcoming

PARENTS' CULTURAL BELIEF SYSTEMS:
THEIR ORIGINS, EXPRESSIONS, AND CONSEQUENCES
Sara Harkness and Charles M. Super, *Editors*

CULTURE AND ATTACHMENT
Perceptions of the Child in Context

ROBIN L. HARWOOD
JOAN G. MILLER
NYDIA LUCCA IRIZARRY

Foreword by Robert A. LeVine

THE GUILFORD PRESS
New York   London

© 1995 The Guilford Press
A Division of Guilford Publications, Inc.
72 Spring Street, New York, NY 10012

Printed in the United States of America

This book is printed on acid-free paper.

Last digit is print number: 9 8 7 6 5 4 3 2

Library of Congress Cataloging-in-Publication Data
Harwood, Robin L.
  Culture and attachment : perceptions of the child
in context / Robin L. Harwood, Joan G. Miller,
Nydia Lucca Irizarry.
      p. cm.
  Includes bibliographical references and index.
  ISBN 0-89862-877-6.—ISBN 1-57230-246-1 (pbk.)
  1. Attachment behavior in children.   2. Attachment
behavior in children—Cross-cultural studies.
3. Interpersonal relations and culture.   4. Interpersonal
relations in children.   I. Miller, Joan G.   II. Irizarry,
Nydia Lucca.   III. Title.
BF723.A75H37   1995
155.4'18—dc20   95-2023
                                                      CIP

*For all of our attachment figures,
past and present*

Foreword

♦

The psychology of attachment grew out of John Bowlby's psychoanalytic studies in Europe and Mary Ainsworth's naturalistic observations in Uganda and Baltimore, but their efforts to transform attachment theory into a universal biopsychology left it strangely detached from local contexts of parental behavior and childhood experiences in human populations. As their context-free approach became dominant in child development research, the need to ground attachment behavior in the cultural symbolism informing parent–child communications and relationships became increasingly apparent and led directly to the research by Robin L. Harwood, Joan G. Miller, and Nydia Lucca Irizarry presented in this book.

The Bowlby–Ainsworth approach to attachment claims to be a "developmental psychiatry" anchored in a biological model and wedded to robust diagnostic procedures for detecting the environmental conditions and behavioral outcomes of normal and abnormal development. Providing an allegedly objective basis for clinical assessment, it replaces moral and ideological judgments of optimal and suboptimal child care with categories validated by empirical research. As part of a science of mental health, attachment research establishes generalizations to guide social policy (e.g., on day care for infants) as well as clinical practice with emotionally disturbed children and adults. This is the appeal of attachment theory to many psychologists and mental health professionals: It is psychoanalysis that has done its homework by building bridges with contemporary biology, creating a vigorous research enterprise, and providing clinicians with useful diagnostic instruments.

The psychology of attachment has its critics, of course, and there are grounds for skepticism concerning its claims and its conception of child development. A central problem is its continued reliance on the distinction between "secure" and "insecure" attachment. The metaphor of emotional security, so clearly a product of 20th-century Euro-American notions of individual needs and interpersonal relations, is a remarkably recent and local concept on which to build a universal model of human development. Yet everything in attachment theory depends on it: All humans become attached to their caregivers, but it is the *quality* of the attachment—that is, its security or insecurity— that provides the basis for estimating mental health risks, and it is as antecedents to secure and insecure forms of attachment that mother– child interactions make their contributions to psychological develop- ment. Neither the possibility that security of attachment was advan- tageous in human evolution, nor its formal operationalization in reli- able assessment procedures eliminates doubt about its status as a universal condition of mental health rather than a culturally contin- gent preference. In other words, judgments of secure and insecure attachment through Ainsworth's Strange Situation procedure, how- ever reliable and theoretically rationalized, might still represent the moral judgments of a particular society at a particular moment in history rather than indicate normality and pathogenesis for all humans at all times.

This suspicion gained support some 10 years ago, when Klaus and Karin Grossmann reported results from their careful replication of Ainsworth's Baltimore study in Bielefeld, North Germany, where a majority of "normal" infants were classified as "insecurely attached." The Grossmanns' suggestion that this departure from American find- ings represented the impact of distinctively German patterns of infant care, without necessarily predicting psychopathology, opened the door for a cultural interpretation of the Strange Situation and called for further evidence on the cultural contexts in which infant–mother at- tachment arises, develops, and manifests itself in behavior.

Research to meet this need has been slow in coming, perhaps because most psychologists interested in attachment would like to believe that they are studying a universal process, whether or not it is the specific one proposed by Bowlby and Ainsworth. Harwood, Miller, and Lucca Irizarry, however, present an alternative view, in which each child is born into a world saturated with cultural meanings that are institutionalized in the values and discourse of a particular commu- nity and reflected in its patterns of social interaction. The develop- ment of the mother–infant relationship is not a biopsychological pro- cess isolated from the cultural values and social patterns of the community; on the contrary, mothers and other caregivers are deeply influenced by culture-specific norms in the preferences that guide their interaction with babies and set goals for their behavioral development. The authors investigate whether mothers of different culturally defined populations vary in their conceptions of desirable interpersonal behavior in situations resembling the Strange Situation as well as more general ones, and their findings in the chapters that follow are full of implications for attachment theory.

To locate a population of mothers differing in their cultural preferences for child behavior and interaction from the American white middle class, Harwood, Miller, and Lucca Irizarry did not have to leave Connecticut, for Puerto Rican mothers there are different in that regard from their Anglo counterparts. In order to avoid confounding cultural background with socioeconomic position, however, they compared mothers on the island of Puerto Rico, where there is a substantial middle-class population, with Anglo mothers (working class as well as middle class) in Connecticut. The findings from their systematic research demonstrate for the first time how culture and social class, separately and together, predict maternal preferences for child behavior both in general and in a simulated Strange Situation. The results presented in this book constitute evidence that the universal repertoire of potential behaviors that infants may manifest in the Strange Situation are subject to culturally specific shaping, such that patterns of attachment behavior classifiable as "secure" can be disapproved in particular cultural settings, while those usually coded as "insecure" may be considered preferable. This raises fundamental questions about the widespread tendency to interpret the secure and insecure attachment categories in terms of universally meaningful mental health risks rather than as individual differences that are differentially interpreted and valued in different groups, *within our own society* as well as elsewhere.

The full force of this evidence can only be appreciated through the words of the Anglo and Puerto Rican mothers themselves, as presented in Chapters Four and Five. Reading their moral evaluations and experiencing the intensity with which they relate ideals of good behavior to their own and others' children makes one wonder how attachment could ever have been treated apart from its cultural context. Harwood, Miller, and Lucca Irizarry have removed the illusion of attachment as a context-free phenomenon and brought it into the field of cultural psychology.

Robert A. LeVine
Harvard University
Graduate School of Education

Acknowledgments

♦

This research was made possible through the support of the National Institutes of Health (Grant No. MH 09911), the National Science Foundation (Grant No. BNS 8903268), and a Research Council Faculty Grant from the University of New Orleans. We are indebted to these institutions for their generous support.

We would like to thank for their assistance the staff of the WIC program of the Hospital of St. Raphael in New Haven, Connecticut, and Angel Pacheco for his assistance in coordinating the data collection in Puerto Rico. For their helpful comments on earlier versions of this book, we thank Klaus Grossmann, Robert Hinde, Axel Schoelmerich, Alan Sroufe, Marinus van IJzendoorn, and the series editors, Sara Harkness and Charlie Super. We also express appreciation to Carolyn Agurcia, Lourdes Aquino, Christa Dalton, Suad Esmail, Melba Gonzolez, Juan Gutierrez, Mark Kenner, Vickie Lucca, Amy Miller, Enrique Morales, Yiba Ng, Lydia Rivas, Steve Ryan, Bryan Sanchez, Nicole Striegel, Roy Tell, Beth Ventura-Cook, and Elba Velazqauez for their assistance with interviewing, translation, and data coding. Finally, our thanks go to Eugenio Ayala, Pam Schulze, and Stephanie Wilson for their help in the preparation of the manuscript.

Contents

♦

CULTURE AND ATTACHMENT

CHAPTER ONE

Attachment Theory and Its Role in the Study of Human Development

♦

In the past two decades, attachment theory, or the study of the bond between an infant and his or her primary caretakers, has emerged as a major domain of inquiry among researchers interested in human development. Its appeal can be attributed to a variety of factors. First, attachment theory possesses a rich and coherent theoretical basis, combining ethological, information-processing, systems control, and psychoanalytic perspectives (Ainsworth, Blehar, Waters, & Wall, 1978; Bowlby, 1969). Second, the study of attachment has been facilitated by the existence of a validated, replicable, and interesting empirical instrument known as the Strange Situation (Ainsworth & Wittig, 1969). Third, attachment theory has proven empirically productive, inasmuch as it has demonstrated the potential for predictive power based on findings of continuity between early quality of attachment and later socioemotional development, as well as the possibility of a primary causal mechanism in caretakers' sensitive, contingent responsiveness to infants' needs. Finally, attachment theory holds the promise of universal applicability among humans as a phylogenetic adaptation of the species.

Given these and other factors, it is no wonder that attachment theory has sparked interest among a wide array of scholars—from investigators seeking to understand basic processes of human development, to clinicians searching for alternative heuristic frameworks;

1

from professionals attempting to formulate public policy regarding the social and emotional health of our nation's children, to researchers struggling with the cultural, historical, and philosophical issues inherent in any definition of optimal mental and emotional health. All these and more have found attachment theory and research a provocative arena for debate. Under what conditions and in what ways can socioemotional functioning in infancy, as indexed by quality of attachment, be said to predict the development of later social and emotional competence? And to what extent can our own ideas of what constitutes "later social and emotional competence" be said to have cross-cultural applicability, even when these ideas are rooted in a vision of universality through phylogenetic adaptation?

This book is not intended to be an exhaustive overview of attachment research. Several book-length reviews have already examined a variety of attachment-related topics, and the interested reader is referred to these (see, e.g., Belsky & Nezworski, 1988; Bretherton & Waters, 1985; Gewirtz & Kurtines, 1991; Gunnar & Sroufe, 1990; Lamb, Thompson, Gardner, & Charnov, 1985; van IJzendoorn, 1990; Parkes & Stevenson-Hinde, 1982; Tavecchio & van IJzendoorn, 1987). Instead, the aim of this book is to focus on one aspect of attachment that has sparked considerable research and debate in the past few years: the role of culture. More specifically, this book explores the rich possibilities inherent in a joint examination of attachment and culture— that is, in the study of attachment from a cultural perspective, and in the study of our cultural constructs from the vantage point of the meanings given to attachment behavior.

For instance, in the past few years several cross-cultural attachment researchers have suggested that although a universal repertoire of attachment behaviors may exist among infants across cultures, the selection, shaping, and interpretation of these behaviors over time appear to be culturally patterned (Bretherton & Waters, 1985; van IJzendoorn, 1990). However, despite a number of empirical studies examining cross-cultural differences in Strange Situation behavior, and despite the frequent use of such key terms as "ecology" and "sociocultural niche," attachment researchers have not explicitly examined different theories of culture or systematically attempted to incorporate these theories into attachment research. Yet such an undertaking has the potential to strengthen our understanding of attachment as a cross-cultural phenomenon through the delineation of coherent conceptual frameworks, which can be used to guide research and help interpret the results of cross-cultural attachment studies. In addition, a closer examination of attachment from a more carefully delineated cultural perspective can sharpen our understanding of the ways in which attachment is both universal and culturally shaped, and thus allow us to evaluate more properly attachment's usefulness as a cross-cultural assessment tool.

Concomitantly, psychologists interested in the larger issues of culture and child development have emphasized the importance of the interactional routines that serve as a social matrix for the acquisition and negotiation of cultural competence (Corsaro & Miller, 1992; Garvey, 1992; Schieffelin & Ochs, 1986). A culturally sensitive study of the meanings attributed to different types of attachment behavior has great potential to enrich this enterprise by its focus on the meaning given to patterns of interaction in infancy. As an age-related and universal phenomenon, attachment behavior and the interactional routines that shape it and give it meaning provide a potentially powerful venue for the study of enculturation in the prelinguistic child.

It would appear, then, that cultural psychology and attachment theory have much to offer each other. It is the joint purpose of this book, therefore, to examine theories of culture and their relevance for attachment, and to examine attachment theory and its relevance for the study of cultural constructs. It seems likely that cross-cultural attachment research can profit from the coherent conceptual framework that a clearer articulation of theories of culture can provide, even as the understanding of cultural constructs different from our own can be enhanced through an examination of perceptions of attachment behavior. In this book, we review two major models of culture and their significance for attachment, and then provide an in-depth discussion of two empirical studies investigating cultural differences in the meanings given to differences in attachment behavior by middle- and working-class Anglo[1] and Puerto Rican mothers.

---

[1]We have chosen the term "Anglo" to describe the white mainland U.S. women of non-Hispanic European ancestry who participated in these studies, for the following reasons: (a) "White U.S. women of non-Hispanic European ancestry" is the most accurate name for this group, but is far too cumbersome for repeated use. (b) Alternative labels such as "Euro-American" or "American" ignore the fact that Puerto Ricans, due to the island's commonwealth status, are not only also of (Hispanic) European ancestry, but are also U.S. citizens. (c) The term "white" is insensitive to the different cultural meanings of race and color in Puerto Rico as compared to the mainland United States. In particular, the racial background of most Puerto Ricans varies widely and in many cases is highly mixed (Spanish, African, and some native island). Thus, two siblings within the same family may differ greatly in their skin

ATTACHMENT THEORY: AN OVERVIEW

Bowlby's Original Formulation

Bowlby (1969) defined attachment as "the bond that ties" the child to his or her primary caretaker, and he considered attachment behaviors to be those behaviors that allow the infant to seek and maintain proximity to this primary attachment figure. Bowlby built his theory of parent–infant attachment on four major theoretical pillars: psychoanalysis, systems control, ethology, and information processing. Each of these influences is evident in attachment theory today.

One of the primary convictions that Bowlby inherited from the psychoanalytic perspective is a belief in the abiding importance of the first 5 years of life for later social and emotional functioning, particularly the importance of the child's first human relationships. However, Bowlby departed from traditional psychoanalytic theory by endorsing a systems control model of human behavior, which he believed was more in accord with principles of modern science than was Freud's model of psychic energy seeking discharge.

In particular, Bowlby argued that instinctive behaviors are mediated by goal-corrected behavioral systems. The most commonly used analogy for a goal-corrected control system is the thermostat, which continually evaluates information regarding temperature. When the temperature falls below a specified set-goal, the thermostat activates the heating system until the temperature is warmed to a point just above the set-goal, at which time the heating system is turned off. Bowlby postulated that many human systems are comparably comprised of various integrated subsystems, which depend on feedback regarding relevant internal and external parameters for their efficient and coordinated operation. For instance, the cardiovascular system of the body operates in such a way that when oxygen demand increases, heart rate and respiration increase also until a physiological balance is achieved between need and intake; when oxygen demand decreases, so do heart rate and respiration; and in this way equilibrium is maintained.

Bowlby hypothesized that a similar process of continual equilibration occurs in the attachment behaviors emitted by infants toward

---

color, but may both be viewed as completely Puerto Rican, and not as "black" or "white" in the racial sense. (d) "Anglo" has a long history of use as a cultural term contrasting the English-speaking Americas with the Spanish-speaking Americas.

their primary caretakers. He considered these attachment behaviors (such as crying, grasping, clinging, reaching, crawling, smiling, and vocalizing) to be part of a behavioral system that has as its set-goal proximity to the caretaker. The attachment system is activated by information concerning the infant's distance from the primary caretaker; when that distance exceeds a certain threshold, the attachment system is activated, and attachment behaviors begin and persist until proximity is regained. Attachment behaviors thus serve to mediate the infant's proximity to the primary caretaker or attachment figure.

Bowlby postulated that the original function of attachment behaviors was protection from predators. Largely on the basis of his ethological observations of attachment in subhuman primates, he argued that human behavioral systems found their beginnings, and therefore their original set-goals and functions, in the environment in which humans originally evolved and to which they became adapted. Because of this, in order to understand a human behavioral system, one must understand the characteristic demands of its "environment of evolutionary adaptedness." Since the primate infant is born in a relatively immature state, it cannot flee unaided from predators or other dangers. Although Bowlby did not conceptualize attachment only in terms of protection from danger, he did emphasize that because attachment behaviors help to maintain the infant's proximity to the parent, they thus served to promote the infant's physical safety and survival in the environment in which humans originally evolved.

According to Bowlby, however, attachment is just one of many behavioral subsystems within the infant. Other important ones include exploration, affiliation, and wariness. The infant's effective functioning depends in part on his or her ability to coordinate these sometimes competing behavioral tendencies into an integrated whole—one that facilitates not only physical survival, but mastery of the environment as well. The coordination of these complex behavioral systems therefore requires the existence of higher processes of integration and control. In other words, it requires the existence of a central information processor that allows the development of an internal working model of the environment and its relevant parameters, as well as of the organism's own capacities to achieve a set-goal under given constraints.

Bowlby's view of the development of an internal working model focused on two key factors: the amount of stress on the attachment system, and the availability of the attachment figure to help alleviate that stress. According to Bowlby, either too much stress or a relatively unavailable attachment figure can, over time, lead to an internal representation of the environment as dangerous and of self and others as ineffective in moderating those dangers; such a representation may leave the child fearful of exploration, uncertain of the availability of safety, doubtful of his or her ability to master environmental demands, and/or distrustful of significant others.

Attachment theory thus returns full circle to central psychoanalytic concerns of the fundamental importance of the child's first relationships for later socioemotional functioning. In particular, if a child repeatedly experiences intense activation of the attachment system coupled with an unavailable attachment figure, then that child is apt to develop over time a representation of himself or herself as someone whose attachment needs are not usually responded to; ultimately, such a child is considered likely to have difficulty expressing needs in situations where it is warranted and perhaps even necessary. In fact, Bowlby suggested that much psychopathology may find its roots in internal working models that are not well adapted to the environmental demands ultimately encountered by the individual.

This, then, was attachment theory as Bowlby initially formulated it: Attachment is a species-typical adaptation that operates as a goal-corrected behavioral system activated by information concerning the proximity–distance threshold from the attachment figure, and having as its function protection from predators. The human infant's attachment history is hypothesized to influence later development in two primary ways. First, early successes in effectively coordinating the attachment subsystem with other behavioral tendencies, such as exploration, affiliation, and wariness, lay a foundation for later healthy functioning, whereas repeated failures predispose an individual toward development along deviant pathways. Second, early experiences of the availability of attachment figures form the basis of an internal working model of relationships, which will serve the child more or less well in meeting the subsequent social and emotional demands of life.

Ainsworth's Formulation

Following Bowlby, Ainsworth similarly defined attachment as "a bond, tie, or enduring relationship between a young child and his or her primary caretaker," and attachment behaviors as those behaviors "through which such a bond first becomes formed and that later serve to mediate the relationship" (Ainsworth et al., 1978, p. 17). Although

Bowlby ultimately articulated a clinically oriented theory of individual differences in attachment behavior (Bowlby, 1973, 1980), it was Ainsworth who made this paradigm explicable and accessible to experimental psychologists through her empirical studies of maternal responsiveness during the first year of life and through the development of a standardized laboratory procedure known as the Strange Situation (Ainsworth, Bell, & Stayton, 1971; Ainsworth et al., 1978; Ainsworth & Wittig, 1969; Stayton & Ainsworth, 1973).

Theoretically, Ainsworth elaborated on Bowlby's view that affect and emotion are part of the organism's appraisal processes. In Bowlby's original formulation, natural danger cues (e.g., noise, strangeness, rapid approach, isolation) activate attachment behavior through the arousal of fear. The arousal of fear and the seeking of safety through retreat to the shelter of a protective attachment figure are part of an animal's basic behavioral equipment and have obvious survival value. Concomitantly, the awareness of potential safety renders a possibly dangerous situation less alarming. For instance, a young animal exploring unfamiliar territory will explore more boldly if it knows that a protective attachment figure is nearby. The removal of the attachment figure augments fear by introducing increased vigilance toward the unfamiliar environment, as well as anxiety over the attachment figure's whereabouts and availability in case of danger; a small child will behave in a similar fashion with his or her primary caretakers.

Ainsworth emphasized that the child's appraisal of the relative presence of threat and security plays a significant role in the behavioral balance of exploration, affiliation, wariness, and attachment that the child demonstrates. A child who has confidence in the attachment figure's availability will feel more free to explore the environment than the child who lacks such confidence. From this perspective, attachment is a goal-corrected system activated by the infant's evaluation of a variety of internal and external parameters that influence the experience of security or insecurity. The set-goal of attachment behaviors is thus broadened to include the infant's subjective sense of security, and the function of attachment behaviors is expanded to embrace a sense of safety, which enables the infant to explore freely and to affiliate with others.

According to this view, the display of attachment behaviors is particularly sensitive to contextual variants that may affect the infant's sense of security, such as setting, familiarity, preceding events, the infant's mood, and developmental level. Over time, however, the infant builds up a stable representation of the attachment figure's general availability and responsiveness despite these variants, and this representation is what is hypothesized to underlie individual differences in attachment behavior (Sroufe & Waters, 1977; Waters, 1978).

The Assessment and Significance of Attachment Behavior

Individual differences in infant attachment behavior are normally assessed when infants are between 12 and 24 months of age, using the standardized laboratory situation devised by Ainsworth and Wittig (1969) and known as the Strange Situation. The Strange Situation consists of seven brief episodes designed to test the infant's ability to use the mother as a secure base for exploring an unfamiliar setting, to respond to the affiliative bids of a stranger, and to recover from the stress caused by separation from the mother in an unfamiliar environment. The Strange Situation thus assesses the balance within the child of four potentially competing behavioral subsystems: exploration, affiliation, wariness, and attachment.

Through a series of four studies using a total of 106 middle-class mother–infant pairs in the Baltimore area, Ainsworth (Ainsworth et al., 1978) developed and confirmed her classification of patterns of Strange Situation behavior into three major groups and eight subgroups. The Group B patterns (consisting of four subgroups: B1, B2, B3, and B4) are generally considered to demonstrate an optimal balance of the organization of behavioral subsystems: Such infants show exploration and affiliation during the preseparation episodes, mild to moderate wariness during separation from the mother, and an ability to be comforted and lack of anger on reunion. In particular, the B1 and B2 patterns (often called the "distal" Bs) combine exploration with relatedness, but generally explore and interact at a greater physical distance from the caretaker; B3 and B4 patterns, in contrast, also combine exploration with relatedness, but tend to explore and interact while maintaining closer proximity to the caretaker.

Infants exhibiting the Group C or "anxious/resistant" patterns (two subgroups, C1 and C2) show little exploration, high distress, and an inability to be comforted by the mother on reunion, with the C1 infant displaying more proximity seeking and contact maintaining than the C2 infant. The Group A or "anxious/avoidant" patterns (two subgroups, A1 and A2) are characterized by low distress during separation and avoidance of proximity to the mother throughout the Strange Situation, with the A1 infant being less likely to physically approach the caretaker than the A2 infant. With the exception of the addition of a Group D or "disorganized/disoriented" attachment pattern said to occur among infants experiencing severe abuse and/or neglect (Main & Solomon, 1986), these eight subclassifications have remained the standard classificatory system in use throughout over 20 years of attachment research.

As Ainsworth conceived it, individual differences in Strange Situation behavior find their roots in maternal sensitivity in responding to infant needs throughout the first year of life (Ainsworth et al., 1971, 1978; Ainsworth & Wittig, 1969; Stayton & Ainsworth, 1973). From this perspective, the infant who has experienced consistent responsiveness will develop a representation of the mother as available to meet his or her needs, and will thus be enabled to use the mother as a secure base for exploration and affiliation in the Strange Situation (the Group B patterns). However, the infant who has experienced inconsistent or inappropriate responsiveness will be uncertain as to the mother's availability and/or caretaking efficacy, leading to reduced exploration and heightened distress in the Strange Situation (Group C behavior). Finally, the infant who experiences rebuff or rejection of his or her needs will develop an apparent deactivation of attachment behaviors directed toward the mother, which, under the moderate stress of the Strange Situation, will take the shape of avoidance of the attachment figure (Group A behavior). This avoidance is considered to be a defensive response that, given the stress of the situation, allows the infant to remain in proximity with the mother without suffering the pain of rebuff, which the infant has come to expect will occur if he or she actively or directly pursues proximity with her (Ainsworth et al., 1978; Main & Weston, 1982; Sroufe & Waters, 1977).

According to this view, then, the three major patterns of attachment behavior represent differing qualities of adaptation; moreover, these differing adaptations are considered to have clear implications for children's current and future socioemotional functioning. In particular, the Group B attachment patterns are held to exemplify optimal negotiation of the primary developmental tasks of infancy, which in turn provide a solid foundation for later healthy functioning. In contrast, the Group A and Group C attachment patterns are viewed as suboptimal organizations of behavior, which lay a foundation for suboptimal outcomes. These foundations are not regarded as *deterministic* of future behavior. However, they are considered to *initiate* developmental trends that make the achievement of later optimal functioning more or less difficult; in this way, early attachment patterns are viewed as either developmental assets or developmental liabilities, which interact with later life circumstances in complex but coherent ways (Belsky & Nezworski, 1988; Main, Kaplan, & Cassidy, 1985; Sroufe, Egeland, & Kreutzer, 1990).

The observant reader will have noted by now several distinct meanings of the term "adaptation" in attachment theory. The failure to distinguish among these has created substantial confusion in the literature (Hinde, 1982; Lamb et al., 1985). In particular, Ainsworth (1984) identified three major definitions or types of adaptation present in attachment theory: (1) phylogenetic adaptation, which corresponds to the phenomenon of attachment itself, hypothesized to have been selected for on the basis of its survival value in the original evolutionary environment; (2) ontogenetic adaptation, which asserts that the behavioral strategies of the human infant are plastic enough to allow for attachment behaviors to develop within, and prove functionally adaptive to, a variety of specific caretaking circumstances; and (3) adaptation in its "developmental mental health" sense—or, rather, the adoption by researchers of a given definition of optimal socioemotional functioning, and the evaluation of specific behaviors in terms of that definition.

In other words, in its *phylogenetic* sense, the formation of an attachment relationship and concomitant behaviors between an infant and his or her primary caretaker(s) is viewed as (and indeed appears to be) a robust phenomenon characteristic of the human species across a wide variety of cultures and caretaking patterns (Lamb et al., 1985; van IJzendoorn & Kroonenberg, 1988). However, individual differences in the patterning of attachment behaviors are regarded as *ontogenetic*, or individual, localized adaptations of the infant to his or her specific caretaking circumstances. Finally, adaptation in its *mental health* sense views certain ontogenetic or individual, localized adaptations as *mal*adaptive when evaluated according to specific criteria of optimal socioemotional functioning; to put it differently, a child may adapt to his or her immediate circumstances, but this adaptation may or may not lay a foundation for optimal development in the mental health sense (Sroufe, 1988). The adaptive significance of attachment behaviors has in this way been expanded to encompass not only a biologically based view of a range of behavioral strategies serving to promote physical survival, but prescriptive definitions of optimal socioemotional functioning as well.

ATTACHMENT AND CROSS-CULTURAL RESEARCH

Given the far-reaching implications of attachment theory for optimal socioemotional development, researchers in the 1980s began to ask whether individual differences in attachment behavior have the same meaning in other cultures as they seem to have in the United States. Study findings indicated that Group A, B, and C attachment classifications were found to occur in somewhat different proportions in other countries and cultures than had been found in dominant U.S. culture. In particular, although Group B classifications were observed to be modal in most cultural groups studied, Group A classifications emerged as relatively more prevalent in Western European countries, whereas Group C classifications were found to be relatively more common in Israel and Japan. In addition, substantial variation in the distribution of the three attachment classifications has been found among infants from differing regional and socioeconomic populations within the same country (Bretherton & Waters, 1985; van IJzendoorn & Kroonenberg, 1988).

These findings led some researchers to begin to re-evaluate the more normative or prescriptive aspects of attachment theory. The implicit normative question took the following form: If, compared to Ainsworth's middle-class Baltimore sample, relatively large proportions of Group A or Group C attachment patterns are obtained among mother–infant pairs from different cultural backgrounds, then how shall we interpret these findings? Shall we say that a large percentage of these children are maladapted in a mental health sense? Although we may, rightly or wrongly, presume to say this about high-risk populations within the United States, we are loath to draw that conclusion regarding middle-class mother–infant pairs living in other countries and cultures. A re-examination of attachment theory's normative claims therefore seemed in order.

It is possible at this point to identify two major approaches to the cross-cultural study of attachment behavior taken by researchers thus far. The first approach has focused on the validity of the Strange Situation, whereas the second, more recent approach focuses on cross-cultural differences in the meanings of attachment behaviors themselves.

Cross-Cultural Validity of the Strange Situation

The question here has often been framed in the following manner: Will infants who rarely experience separation from their mothers (such as Japanese infants), or who have infrequent contact with unfamiliar people (such as kibbutz-reared Israeli infants), perceive the Strange Situation to be as stressful as do middle-class U.S. infants? If not, how can the Strange Situation be modified for use with different cultural groups, in order to insure equivalence of its emotional meaning to the infants involved, and therefore universality of the meaning of the behaviors displayed (Nakagawa, Lamb, & Miyake, 1988; Sagi, 1990; Takahashi, 1986, 1990)?

In general, it appears that caretaking circumstances do have an impact on the perceived stressfulness of the Strange Situation as a whole (although it must be noted that Sagi, van IJzendoorn, & Koren-Karie, 1991, conclude that the appraisal of the *preseparation* episodes is similar across a wide variety of cultures). In addition, the procedure itself can be modified for use with different sociocultural groups in such a way as to produce classification distributions comparable to those obtained by Ainsworth in her Baltimore samples. On the other hand, some of these modifications to the Strange Situation (e.g., eradicating the infant-alone episode) leave one wondering whether the infants in question are indeed experiencing comparable situations.

Although Sagi and his colleagues (Oppenheim, Sagi, & Lamb, 1988; Sagi et al., 1991) conclude that the predictive power of the Strange Situation is robust with regard to procedural variations, we must nonetheless ask this question: Does the Strange Situation become at some point a different as opposed to a modified procedure? And, if this is so, then are we only masking what may be real sociocultural differences? It may be that in attempting to make the perceived stressfulness of the Strange Situation equivalent across sociocultural settings, we are obscuring important differences in the cultural meanings ascribed to various attachment behaviors in the first place. To put it differently, in focusing on the production of similar behaviors, we have emphasized the capacity for a universal repertoire of attachment behaviors. However, it may be time to give more attention to culturally differentiated meanings of attachment behavior.

For example, we may note that laughter is a common phenomenon among humans; we may even hypothesize that it is a universal phenomenon connoting levity. Let's say that in order to test our hypothesis, we construct a joke and tell it to participants in several cultures. We discover that the joke results in the same level of laughter in all cultural contexts only when the joke has been modified in a variety of ways. We conclude that laughter occurs universally among humans, and that joke telling is a robust predictor of laughter. However, by having to modify our stimulus material, we also acknowledge that the circumstances under which laughter occurs are culturally variable. Moreover, the normative expression of laughter as a response to our joke varies as well, with a hearty guffaw being considered appropriate in one setting, and a quiet chuckle in another. We may go further and postulate that learning to guffaw as opposed to chuckle in one circumstance and not another is inherent in the process of becoming a socially competent member of a specific culture. By continually modifying our joke so that it produces, say, a chuckle as the normative response, we have indeed demonstrated that chuckles may exist as part of a universal human repertoire. But in so doing, we have obscured the particular meanings given to laughter and joke telling among a given group of people, and it is the knowledge of *particular* meanings—knowing when and where to laugh, to cry, to be afraid, and to seek comfort—that ultimately defines social competence.

Contextualized Meaning of Attachment Behaviors

Several cross-cultural attachment researchers have thus suggested a move beyond "the search for a so-called culture-free test . . . to [a] search for differences in outcome in different cultures" (van IJzendoorn, 1990, p. 7). Or, as K. E. Grossmann and Grossmann (1990) put it: "The main issue is whether the different attachment strategies observed may be differentially adaptive in different cultures. . . . It may well be that behavior strategies are universal, but that the relevance for them may be culture-specific" (p. 37). In a similar vein, Sagi (1990) notes that "we can conclude that attachment theory is useful in the broader sense but always must be applied within the context of cultural idiosyncrasies. Or, to state the case from a universalistic point of view, the repertoire of attachment behaviors is similar across countries, but the selection of these behaviors is culturally specific" (p. 19).

What these investigators are suggesting is that cross-cultural attachment research may now be at the point of moving beyond the search for universals to a more careful study of the contextualized meaning of attachment behavior, its antecedents, and its consequences. This does not mean that the search for universals has failed. On the contrary, it seems clear that, except in the most extreme cases of severe neglect, all infants become attached to their primary caretakers; that they exhibit a specifiable range of attachment behaviors toward their caretakers under conditions of sufficient stress; and that Group B attachment patterns in particular appear to be modal in most cultural contexts studied thus far (Lamb et al., 1985; van IJzendoorn, 1990). However, what remains largely unexamined is the role that cultural values and norms play—not only in what Sagi (1990) terms the culturally specific selection of particular attachment behaviors, but also in our very definition of what constitutes desirable or optimal socioemotional outcomes.

Several researchers have suggested that the observed variation in the distribution of infants across the three major attachment classifications may reflect, in part, differences in cultural meaning systems and concomitant socialization patterns (van IJzendoorn, 1990).[2] K. Grossmann, Grossmann, Spangler, Suess, and Unzner (1985), for example, suggested that the high percentage of Group A attachments in their north German sample may reflect a cultural preference for early independence training among north German mothers. Similarly, Miyake, Chen, and Campos (1985) offered the possibility that the high percentage of Group C infants in their Japanese sample may be attributable in part to aspects of Japanese society that encourage the child's emotional interdependence on family members (*amae*), and thus render his or her experience of separation from the mother extremely rare.

From this perspective, the mental health meanings of certain behaviors must be examined in the context of larger environmental demands, as well as differences in parental behaviors and socialization goals. Ontogenetic adaptations may have culturally specific relevance, and the meanings of those adaptations can therefore be evaluated only in the context of their fit with the larger family and sociocultural settings. For instance, in Japan a greater valuing of emotional interdependence is associated with limited separation experiences, therefore

---

[2]It should be noted that recent work examining communal versus family sleeping arrangements among Israeli kibbutzim (Sagi, van IJzendoorn, Aviezer, Donnell, & Mayseless, 1994) suggests that communal sleeping, more than other cultural factors associated with Israeli society, appears to be responsible for the high incidence of Group C attachment relationships among kibbutzim infants.

heightening the distress experienced by many Japanese infants in the Strange Situation. However, because the family environment of these infants is in accord with the values and expectations of the larger sociocultural setting, the mental health implications of their heightened distress is not the same as it would be in dominant U.S. culture, which values the cultivation of independence.

Cultural meaning systems, then, influence the behavioral patterns that infants may show in the Strange Situation. There is another level, however, at which cross-cultural differences in the meaning of attachment behavior may arise: In particular, they may arise at the more symbolic level of the very constructs we use to describe what constitutes desirable socioemotional functioning. According to this view, focus shifts from the relative incidence of specific behaviors to the interrelationships of the meanings given to all behaviors. For example, cultural values and childcare arrangements may produce a higher incidence of distress among Japanese infants exposed to an unmodified Strange Situation, and the meaning of that heightened distress is rightly examined only in the context of the larger sociocultural setting in which it occurs. However, cultural meaning systems extend beyond specific child care arrangements to encompass culturally constituted conceptions of the self, others, and the world they inhabit. From this perspective, the focus of attention is no longer whether Japanese babies look more like Group C babies in an unmodified Strange Situation, or more like Group B babies in a modified procedure. Instead, the emphasis shifts to the central cultural constructs (e.g., *amae* or emotional interdependence) that inform the behaviors in question, and that interrelate Strange Situation behaviors to patterns of behavior in other aspects of life. The meaning of attachment behavior can thus be considered part of a culturally constructed web of meanings regarding the relationship of self to other. Japanese toddlers, like their U.S. counterparts, are involved in a lifelong process of learning (or failing to learn) what it means to be competent members of their social group; the optimal balance of autonomy and relatedness, as well as appropriate displays of curiosity, affiliation, and comfort seeking, is part of that web of meaning. In order, then, to begin to understand the culturally contextualized meaning of attachment behavior, it is necessary to begin to understand the cultural constructs that inform the behaviors observed. Before we examine more carefully the relevance of cultural constructs for attachment, it is necessary to consider the role of culturally desirable endpoints in developmental theory.

Culture and Desirable Developmental Endpoints

What Constitutes a Desirable Endpoint?

In recent years, several researchers have commented on the role that cultural values play in our definition of what constitutes optimal development. In 1979, Kessen suggested that child psychology "is itself a peculiar cultural invention that moves with the tidal sweeps of the larger culture in ways that we understand at best dimly and often ignore" (p. 815). Bruner (1986) similarly commented that "in principle theories of human development constitute . . . a science whose intrinsic object is not simply to describe but to prescribe alternative optimal ways of achieving certain outcomes. . . . we create an implicit world such as we think one *ought* to be" (pp. 20–21). Wartofsky (1986) likewise noted that "theories of development [are] affected by [*sic*] the whole range of [social, political, and cultural] artifacts which, in any given period, come to define the range and character of the accepted or approved modes of child activity or of child development" (p. 125). S. White (1983, p. 74) concludes that "the idea of development in developmental psychology is a systematic idea, but it is very likely to be treated as an ethical idea."

In short, the idea of development in its systematic sense presumes by definition an end state toward which the organism is developing (Laboratory of Comparative Human Cognition, 1983; S. White, 1983). Thus, for example, Piaget conceived of the capacity for formal operational thinking as the end state of cognitive development; Kohlberg posited principled moral thinking to be the ultimate goal of moral development; Margaret Mahler viewed psychological development as a process of separation–individuation, with emotional object constancy as its aim; Freud considered the psychological endpoint of development to be a healthy Oedipal resolution, which he viewed as essential to the fully realized capacity "to work and to love" in adulthood. Each of these theories specified an endpoint toward which the development of the individual (if not the entire species) should strive. Each of these theories has also faced modification and revision in light of cross-cultural research, which has suggested that the posited end state is based on a culturally specific vision of what constitutes the ultimate good.

This is not to say that the specification of endpoints somehow implies an "unscientific" subjective bias, which should be eliminated from developmental theorizing in favor of more "objective" criteria. On the contrary, several researchers have argued that the exercise of value-based choices regarding what is deemed more or less optimal in human behavior may be part and parcel not only of developmental theory properly conceived, but also of the entire psychological enterprise (Howard, 1985; Scarr, 1985; Schwartz, 1990). Moreover, self-conscious reflection on the norms and values that inevitably underlie our theories may enable us to construct more wisely the good that we wish for ourselves and our children. As Bruner (1986) notes: "Without explicit value presuppositions, we will fall into the habit of forming implicit ones and lose such power as we might have either in furthering or opposing the values of the culture in which we find ourselves" (p. 27). As psychologists interested in human development, then, we have the responsibility to engage in self-criticism of our own normative proposals (Marcus & Fischer, 1986; Wartofsky, 1986).

Attachment, Culture, and Desirable Endpoints

Inasmuch as attachment theory constitutes a normative developmental model—inasmuch as it makes claims regarding not only what is *now*, but what is likely to *become*, more or less "optimal" socioemotional functioning—then attachment theory makes claims regarding desirable endpoints. As such, it is open to the same criticisms (and potentially to the same richness) that has characterized other developmental theories. In particular, attachment theorists have characterized the Group B attachment patterns as desirable, in that these children are more likely at later preschool ages to display autonomy, curiosity, ego resilience, positive exploration, enthusiasm, persistence in problem solving, and high self-esteem (Arend, Gove, & Sroufe, 1979; Matas, Arend, & Sroufe, 1978; Sroufe, Fox, & Pancake, 1983), as well as sociability, cooperation, compliance with adult directives, empathy, positive affect, and competence in the peer group (LaFreniere & Sroufe, 1985; Londerville & Main, 1981; Waters, Wippman, & Sroufe, 1979).

In other words, the Group B attachment pattern is associated with a balance of autonomy and relatedness that we consider optimal in modern U.S. society. It is likely, however, that the same attachment pattern would be interpreted differently, given a different meaning system. For instance, a middle-class Anglo mother from the mainland United States may watch a toddler playing happily and quietly in the preseparation episode of the Strange Situation and interpret this as demonstrating curiosity, independence, and a sense of inner security—signs that the infant is developing a positive sense of self. In contrast, a middle-class Puerto Rican mother in Puerto Rico may watch the same infant and see instead a calmness and willingness to engage with the environment—qualities suggesting that the child is *educado* or well-taught/teachable, and will become respectfully attentive to others. In this way, the study of attachment is a potentially rich source for understanding the culturally prescribed meanings given to patterns of social and emotional behavior throughout life.

It may be that Group B attachment behavior is associated with a variety of positively valued characteristics across many cultures. The fact that Group B attachments have been found to be modal in most cultural groups studied thus far lends some weight to this claim (although this does not invalidate the possibility that in some circumstances Group A or Group C attachments may fit children to grow up into adults who best meet the cultural norms; see deVries, 1984; Hinde, 1982). However, of major importance for the study of culture and ultimately for a sensitive cross-cultural analysis of attachment itself is the *meaning* given to optimal patterns of attachment behavior by different sociocultural groups. Through studying these meanings, we can gain a better understanding of cultural definitions of social competence, and the ways in which those definitions organize parent–infant interactional routines from infancy onwards. We examine this in more depth in the next chapter, in our discussion of attachment and theories of culture.

CHAPTER TWO

Child Development
and Theories of Culture

◆

We have noted in Chapter One that despite a number of empirical studies examining cross-cultural differences in Strange Situation behavior, and despite the use of such key terms as "ecology" and "sociocultural niche," attachment researchers have not explicitly examined different theories of culture or systematically attempted to incorporate these theories into attachment research. Yet progress in cross-cultural attachment research may depend in part on the explicit articulation of theoretical models of culture, for it is only through such self-conscious reflection that we can systematically generate conceptual frameworks within which to examine and understand our cross-cultural findings. In this chapter, we briefly examine the history of two broad theoretical approaches to the study of culture, and discuss some of their current implications for cross-cultural attachment research.

HISTORICAL OVERVIEW OF
CULTURAL ADAPTATIONISM

Origins of the Culture and Personality Movement

Historically, both cultural anthropology and developmental psychology emerged from the progressive-developmental paradigm. Although its origins are traceable as far back as the ancient Greeks (Lovejoy, 1936), this paradigm saw perhaps its fullest flowering in the 19th-century evolutionist writings of such thinkers as Spencer, Haeckel, Romanes, Preyer, Morgan, Tylor, and Frazer (Morss, 1990; Stocking, 1984; S. White, 1983). Based on non-Darwinian evolutionary speculation, as well as on a misreading of Darwinian evolutionary theory itself, the progressive-developmental paradigm maintained that development consists of an orderly sequence of changes that are parallel across the individual, the history of civilization, and the course of evolution itself.

This paradigm ceased to be dominant in the nascent field of cultural anthropology in the early decades of the 20th century, in part because of post-World War I disillusionment with the idea that Western civilization is self-evidently superior, and in part because of the rise of structural–functional approaches to the study of human society (e.g., Durkheim, Malinowski, Radcliffe-Brown). The field of child psychology, on the other hand, took a somewhat different historical course from its sister field of cultural anthropology, in that the search for universal, orderly, and sequential stages of development remained a more central and paradigmatically dominant concern (e.g., Freud, Werner, Piaget).

The *cultural* study of the child, however, emerged from within the Malinowskian school of functionalism in anthropology, most particularly through the writings of Margaret Mead (1928) and Ruth Benedict (1934), who are generally credited with founding the "culture and personality" movement—a movement whose long dominance in cross-cultural child psychology is still felt (e.g., see Segall, Dasen, Berry, & Poortinga, 1990). In its original formulation, the culture and personality movement maintained that culturally specific child-rearing practices lead to modal or national personality types, which in turn influence societal patterns and institutions. For instance, harsh toilet training practices by most parents within a given group could be hypothesized to lead to a modal personality type in which adults mask underlying hostility with an outwardly submissive attitude toward authority; such explanations were offered around the time of World War II as a rationale for the societal readiness of the German people to embrace the Nazi movement (see Sargent & Smith, 1949). However, the search to delineate national personality configurations ended ultimately in failure. This failure, combined with the rise of the ecosystem concept in anthropology (Odum, 1953; Steward, 1955), led to a revision of the culture and personality school of thought (see Hsu, 1961).

Cultural Adaptationism

The ecosystem concept emphasized that living organisms and their environment are inseparably interrelated, and it defined the ecological niche as the position of an organism within its ecosystem resulting from the organism's structural adaptations and behaviors (Odum, 1953). In the later formulation of the culture and personality school, the ecosystem model was combined with elements of the original culture and personality movement; it is this later formulation that gained ascendancy in the cross-cultural study of the child, reaching perhaps its fullest elaboration in the works of Whiting (J. W. M. Whiting, 1961, 1977; B. B. Whiting & Whiting, 1975) and the early work of LeVine (1973). This approach, which we have chosen to call "cultural adaptationism"[1] after Keesing (1981), provided psychologists with a powerful theoretical tool for understanding child behavior in cross-cultural context. It should be noted that a model based more purely on the concept of the ecosystem without benefit of the culture and personality movement was also propounded by Barker and Gump (1964) and Bronfenbrenner (1977), and it is thus common for child development researchers to make reference to certain aspects of an ecosystem model without adopting all of the tenets of cultural adaptationism (e.g., Garbarino, 1990; Spencer & Markstrom-Adams, 1990).

However, the continued influence of cultural adaptationism among psychologists interested in the cultural study of the child is evident to this day (see Ogbu, 1981; Segall et al., 1990). For instance, the *Child Development* special issue on minority children (April 1990) contained five theoretically oriented review articles; three of the five appealed to key elements of what we are calling "cultural adaptationism" for understanding the development of minority children. For

---

[1]We are choosing to limit our discussion of cultural adaptationism to those approaches that have most directly influenced theories of culture in the study of child psychology. However, we would be remiss if we did not mention that theoretical affinities are generally agreed to exist (Keesing, 1981; Orlove, 1980) between the ecological approaches exemplified by Steward (1955) and the cultural-evolutionary perspective typified by L. A. White (1959). It must also be noted that much of the discussion that follows is not relevant to more contemporary, processual manifestations of this approach (e.g., Boyd & Richerson, 1985). Unfortunately, this latter approach has only just begun to have an impact on child development theorizing (see Tomasello, Kruger, & Ratner, 1993); we therefore confine our discussion to the approach that has had the largest impact on cross-cultural research in child psychology.

pedagogical purposes, therefore, despite the fact that researchers some-times focus only on the ecosystem concept, we concentrate our dis-cussion on cultural adaptationism in its fully elaborated form.

Cultural adaptationism views the socializing context of the child as an ecosystem in which the physical environment, modes of produc-tion, social organization, and belief systems are all viewed as func-tionally interdependent and coexisting in an adaptive equilibrium (see Segall et al., 1990; J. W. M. Whiting, 1961). Moreover, the first link in the adaptationist chain is generally held to be the physical environ-ment and its related economy and modes of production. Personality traits, behavioral characteristics, and attitudes that promote the con-tinued harmony of the ecosystem are selected for in the process of cultural transmission. Culture itself is ultimately defined as socially transmitted behaviors which are adaptive to an environment common to a specific group of people (Keesing, 1981). For instance, in their classic study, Barry, Child, and Bacon (1959), influenced by Steward's (1955) work on cultural ecology, hypothesized that societies with low accumulation of food resources would emphasize the development of individualism, assertiveness, and initiative, whereas societies with high accumulation of food resources would seek to instill conscientious-ness and compliance in their children. From this perspective, adult personality plays a functional role in relation to the economy of the society, and the goal of child training is to produce personality traits most adaptive to the given society's economic needs and demands (see B. B. Whiting & Whiting, 1975).[2]

More recently, B. B. Whiting and Edwards (1988) have continued to elaborate a cultural-adaptationist approach to the cross-cultural study of the child. In particular, they describe different maternal pro-files in six cultures (Liberia, Kenya, India, the Philippines, Mexico, and the United States), and relate differential emphases on maternal control, training, and sociability to ecological constraints within the mothers' lives. For example, a strong emphasis on training children to do specific household chores is held to be associated with circum-stances in which the mother is the major producer of food for the family, and thus has a workload extending beyond housework and

[2]It is also worth noting that Malinowski's own interest in Freud (Malinowksi, 1927) laid a foundation within the Culture and Personality movement for a psychoanalytic approach to the study of the ecosystem. Freudian theory thus provided a framework for understanding the mechanisms by which child-rearing practices, adult personal-ity, and a society's projective systems were all functionally interrelated (see Hsu, 1961; J. W. M. Whiting, 1961).

child care; this greater workload necessitates a higher proportion of household help from the children, and so leads to a greater emphasis on training. Similarly, the authors relate the relatively strong emphasis on sociable mother–child interactions in the United States to the fact that U.S. mothers are more likely to be residentially isolated and spending their days mostly in the company of young children. Whiting and Edwards diverge somewhat from the classic adaptationist model, in that they focus on the ways in which cultures place children of different ages and genders in different settings, thus providing them with opportunities to learn and practice different skills. However, the basic focus on finding functional relationships among subsistence patterns, parental practices, and socialization goals remains unchanged.

Although attachment researchers have not generally articulated a theory of culture on which to base their cross-cultural investigations, there has been a tendency to assume some of the basic tenets of the cultural-adaptationist approach. This has been evident in (1) assertions regarding presumed functional interrelationships among specific child-rearing practices, socialization goals, environmental variables, and attachment outcomes; (2) implicit suppositions that these elements should bear some lawful relationship to one another; (3) tentative speculation that cultural values (e.g., "independence" or "obedience") may lead to specific child-rearing practices that seek to form individual adult personalities in keeping with the cultural or national ideal (see the closing discussion in Hinde & Stevenson-Hinde, 1990); and (4) finally, the compatibility of an adaptationist approach with attachment theory's own rootedness in ethology, evolutionary theory, and psychoanalytic thought.

As an approach, then, cultural adaptationism has tended to appeal to child psychologists in general and to attachment researchers in particular for perhaps two primary reasons. First, because of its historical theoretical emphasis on processes rooted in evolutionary theory (in particular, natural selection and organismic adaptation), it has seemed a natural ally for a subdiscipline that traces its lineage to Darwin and 19th-century theories of progressive development (see Kessen, 1965; Mandelbaum, 1971; S. White, 1983). Bowlby's own indebtedness to evolutionary theory is also apparent, thus solidifying the foundation for the use of an adaptationist approach to the study of culture by attachment researchers. Second, the natural science model implicit in an adaptationist approach is attractive to researchers who hope to find lawful relationships among environmental variables, child-rearing practices, and developmental outcomes.

HISTORICAL AND THEORETICAL OVERVIEW OF SYMBOLIC APPROACHES

General Concerns

There is a second major approach to the study of culture, which attachment theorists may find a useful supplement to elements drawn from cultural adaptationism. Strictly speaking, this second theoretical framework is not an "approach" so much as it is a *set* of approaches diverse in their particulars, which nonetheless share certain fundamental tenets regarding the centrality of symbolic meaning systems for understanding and interpreting human behavior. Although anthropological and psychological approaches drawing upon the idea of the ecosystem are also diverse in their particulars, the dominance within cross-cultural psychology of the culture and personality movement makes it easier to label and articulate a single paradigm characterizing this school of thought and its impact on child development research.

Unfortunately, the lack of dominance of any one paradigm renders the very act of labeling our second set of approaches a difficult one; however, given the shared importance these approaches assign to symbolic meaning systems and to the interpretation of human behavior, we have chosen to include them under the rubric of "symbolic" approaches. Despite their diversity, symbolic approaches to the social sciences generally share the assumption that human beings construct meaning through their cultural symbol systems, with language being one of culture's most powerful symbol systems. Many of these approaches go on to assert that this construction occurs within a matrix of social interaction (e.g., Berger & Luckmann, 1966; Gumperz & Hymes, 1986; Schieffelin & Ochs, 1986; Vygotsky, 1978).

Difficulties in characterizing symbolic approaches are further compounded by the frequent equation of the theory underlying symbolic approaches with the qualitative methodologies generally associated with them. On a theoretical level, symbolic approaches seek to understand culturally constituted meaning systems, but this goal may be pursued through a variety of methodologies, both qualitative and quantitative. On a methodological level, symbolic approaches are historically associated with qualitative methodologies (e.g., anthropological field study or textual analysis) rather than quantitative ones. The frequent equation of symbolic theories with qualitative methodologies alone has rendered these approaches too often opaque to psychologists concerned with conventional empirical standards of methodological rigor.

However, it is our contention that a distinction between the symbolic theoretical component and the qualitative methodological component of this set of approaches may serve to invigorate research in this area through a partial decoupling of theory and methodology. For instance, it may be true that qualitative data (e.g., data based on open-ended interviews, as opposed to more quantitative or closed assessments) are part of many symbolic approaches to the study of culture; however, qualitative data are themselves neutral to the type of methodology employed to analyze them. One can analyze qualitative data using either traditional interpretive (e.g., ethnography and textual or conversational analysis) or quantitative methodologies, or some combination of the two; however, the standards of methodological rigor applied in each case will be relative to the type of methodology employed.

Historical Overview

Although symbolic approaches have represented a less dominant perspective in mainstream psychology, their historical roots are no less long and no less illustrious than those of the progressive-developmental paradigm. The term "hermeneutics," or the theory of interpretation, derives from the Greeks, and the practice of hermeneutics existed in Germany as a method of Biblical study from the time of the Protestant Reformation onward. In 1829, Schleiermacher systematized the hermeneutic method, defining it as the psychological–historical reconstruction of the meaning of a text, and raising the status of what was a collection of ad hoc precepts and practices to that of a critical theory of knowledge (Ermarth, 1978). This hermeneutic tradition was translated into a historic methodology by Wilhelm Dilthey (1883–1893/1985).

Dilthey's thought existed in and reflects the creative tension that characterized 19th-century European philosophy. The century had begun with the rise and subsequent fall of Kantian and Hegelian idealism, only to find itself entrenched in its latter half in the positivism first expounded by Comte and Mill. In the midst of an intellectual battleground that pitted the primacy of sense data against the priority of the mind's own categories of knowing, Dilthey sought a middle ground, arguing that through the hermeneutic process it is possible,

through a series of self-reflective approximations, to elevate understanding (*Verstehen*) in the human sciences toward general validity
by seeking objectified meanings within a coherence of contexts
(Ermarth, 1978). Dilthey believed that life is a constant pattern of
interpretive efforts based on concrete human experiences. However,
inasmuch as higher forms of human understanding entail increasingly
complex patterns of meaning, Dilthey considered that the proper study
of the human sciences is thus to seek to understand those patterns of
meaning. He adopted the term *Geisteswissenschaften* for his approach—
a term that first received currency in 1849 with the translation into
German of J. S. Mill's *System of Logic*. Although the word was originally used to translate the expression "moral sciences," Dilthey broadened the scope of *Geisteswissenschaften* to such an extent that it is
today generally translated into English as "human sciences," the proper
scope of which is purported to be the understanding of human conduct
(Alexander & Seidman, 1990). Twentieth-century proponents of a
hermeneutic approach to the social sciences have included Gadamer
(1975) and Ricoeur (1978).

As Cahan and White (1992) describe for us, the search for a science of human nature concerned with meaning as well as lawful behavior has had advocates as far back as the founders of positivism
and empiricism themselves, Comte and Mill. However, the positivist
and empiricist goals and methods that gave birth to modern psychology were initially unable to include the more "purposive" aspects of
human nature within their proper dominion. Nonetheless, the recognition of and search for appropriate methods to study a purposive
psychology has continued in psychology throughout the 20th century,
from Wundt, Dewey (Cahan, 1992), and G. H. Mead to recent inter-
preters of Vygotsky (Cole, 1985; Wertsch, 1985).

In contemporary social theory, three streams of thought have
come together with what might loosely be called the *Geisteswissenschaften* tradition to form the basis of symbolic approaches in the social
sciences (see Alexander & Seidman, 1990; Giddens, 1976, 1987):
(1) the influence of the post-Wittgensteinian movement in U.S. and
British philosophy (e.g., Austin, 1975; Winch, 1958), which sought
to understand the process by which social relationships are constituted
through shared norms regarding how to speak and behave properly
and meaningfully within a given speech community; (2) the phenomenological tradition represented by Husserl (1960) and Schutz (1967),
which maintained that human intentionality involves an act of idea-
tion distinct from and not reducible to the object of attention itself;

and (3) the rise of semiotics (e.g., Derrida, 1978; Saussure, 1974), which emphasized both the centrality of language for philosophy and social theory, and the essentially arbitrary nature of the sign symbols that constitute language. Symbolic approaches to the social sciences have included, among others, the symbolic interactionism of G. H. Mead (1934; Blumer, 1987); the "interactionism" of sociolinguistics (Gumperz & Hymes, 1986) and ethnomethodology (Garfinkel, 1967); the postmodern schools of thought in cultural anthropology (Clifford, 1986; Manganaro, 1990); the phenomenological perspective of Berger and Luckmann (1966); the social constructionism articulated in recent years in psychology (Shweder, 1990); the sociohistorical position of Vygotsky (1978); the linguistic method of Lakoff (Lakoff & Johnson, 1980); the more cognitive approaches of Bruner (1990) and D'Andrade (D'Andrade & Strauss, 1992); and the interactional view of socialization outlined by Schieffelin and Ochs (1986).

Theoretical Overview

On a methodological level, symbolic approaches generally maintain that social science is unlike natural science, inasmuch as it involves the interpretation of contextually meaningful human behavior rather than the discovery of universal laws. As Little (1991) observes: "To provide a satisfactory analysis of a given social phenomenon, it is necessary to arrive at an interpretation of the meanings that agents within that culture assign to their actions and social relations" (p. 69). Others have gone on to maintain that the study of human behavior cannot advance further without a return to the study of its *meaning* (see Fiske & Shweder, 1986).

On a theoretical level, symbolic approaches in the social sciences generally seek to understand the relationship between person and environment by viewing them as coconstitutive or mutually emergent (Geertz, 1973; Gergen, 1985). As Shweder (1990, p. 2) notes: "[N]o sociocultural environment exists or has identity independent of the way human beings seize meanings and resources from it, while every human being has her or his subjectivity and mental life altered through the process of seizing meanings and resources from some sociocultural environment and using them."

From this perspective, individuals and society construct one another. Moreover, the medium through which this coconstruction largely occurs is the language of a given speech community (Gumperz,

1972). Humans construct meaning through their cultural symbol systems, and language is one of culture's most powerful symbol systems; it is the means through which most of culture is learned and communicated. However, language is viewed not as an individual psychological capacity, but rather as the shared understandings and activities of persons engaged in social interactions with one another (Gergen, 1985). In other words, individual vocal and verbal activities do not exist independently of the shared and established codes of meaning that create them (Geertz, 1973). Instead, linguistic acts are socially organized and embedded in sociocultural systems of meaning, just as those same meaning systems are continually either reinforced, negotiated, or transformed by social interactants (Gumperz, 1982; Shweder, 1990). The unit of description is thus a social rather than a linguistic entity, and is defined as a community of people who share knowledge of rules and norms for the conduct and interpretation of speech. To study culture, then, is to study shared codes of meaning (Geertz, 1973; Gumperz, 1972), and to study the individual in culture may thus involve an examination of culturally constituted or shared psychological processes.

A major characteristic of language or speech as shared activity is its rule-governed nature (Searle, 1972). The most common analogies for this approach to culture are socially constituted, rule-governed games such as baseball, chess, or cricket. Just as in a game, social interactants must share an understanding of the norms and rules governing conduct in order for a given interaction to go smoothly; moreover, shared understandings are continually negotiated during the course of an interaction. According to Gumperz and Hymes (1986), communication thus does not proceed according to fixed rules. Instead, it is a two-step process in which a given speaker "first takes in stimuli from the outside environment, evaluating and selecting from among them in the light of his own cultural background, personal history, and what he knows about his interlocutors. He then decides on the norms that apply to the situation at hand" (p. 15). From this description, it is evident that a social interactant must know which set of rules to invoke and select from. In addition, interactants actively negotiate and create shared meanings during the course of an interaction, even as their choices reflect the constraints of their culturally available models.

It is also evident that the norms governing interactions will vary from context to context and from culture to culture (Cole, 1983; Gumperz, 1982). In order to become socially competent, then, a child must become proficient in the cultural norms that govern conduct and its evaluation among members of a given speech community (Laboratory of Comparative Human Cognition, 1983; Schieffelin & Ochs, 1986). Through the process of socialization, individuals become skilled in using culturally available models to construct and interpret their experience; moreover, individuals may transform these models in unexpected ways, thus highlighting both the active role of the individual in creating and recreating culture, and the dynamic nature of culture itself. Through everyday social interactions with adults and older children, young children abstract interactional norms and gain culture- and context-specific understandings and social competencies. Socialization is thus context-specific, and views the child as an active organizer of the rule-governed understandings to be abstracted from everyday social interactions. From this standpoint, culture is "contested, temporal, and emergent" (Clifford, 1986, p. 19); it "is concerned with what Kenneth Burke called 'strategies for the encompassing of situations' . . . [and] is less about how to speak well than about how to speak at all, and to act meaningfully, in the world of public cultural symbols" (Clifford, 1986, pp. 11–12). A symbolic cultural approach to the psychological study of the individual may thus involve an examination of culturally constituted psychological processes, including culturally shared cognitive models and meaning systems.

THEORETICAL APPROACHES TO THE STUDY OF CULTURE AND ATTACHMENT

As this overview of theories of culture has shown, there are at least two major models one may draw from when approaching cross-cultural attachment research: cultural adaptationism and a symbolic approach. These models are not necessarily mutually exclusive, and may be used in a complementary fashion to understand different aspects of the child in context.

Cultural Adaptationism

Cultural adaptationism traces its theoretical roots in part to the progressive-developmental paradigm, but that heritage is strongly attenuated and exists now primarily through its appeal to ethological research, ecology, and the biological evolution of the human species.

Emphasis is placed on the adaptation of the infant to the ecosystem of the child-rearing environment. In particular, this perspective maintains that different qualities of attachment reflect differing adaptations to the immediate caretaking environment, and that differential frequencies of Group A, B, and C attachment patterns may be obtained across groups or cultures, because of differences in caretaking styles and socialization goals. From this standpoint, the mental health meanings of individual differences in attachment behavior may remain an open question. As K. E. Grossmann and Grossmann (1990) and Sagi (1990) have observed, specific strategies are selected from the apparently universal repertoire of attachment behaviors in the context of specific cultural requirements, and thus their adaptive consequences can be evaluated only within that same context. Therefore, if a relatively large percentage of Group A or Group C attachments is obtained, then the mental health consequences of this finding can be considered only with reference to the socialization goals and practices of the sociocultural setting in question.

Symbolic Approach

According to a symbolic approach, the parent–infant relationship represents an important matrix in which the child continually constructs and negotiates meanings. Whereas the adaptationist approach emphasizes the lawful relations obtained between environmental and behavioral variables, the symbolic approach treats culture as a system of meaning not explicable merely in terms of functional adaptation to the environment. According to this view, optimal mental health represents the child's ability to negotiate successfully the social demands of culturally salient settings. Since salient settings and their successful negotiation are defined culturally, optimal mental health becomes, in part, by definition a cultural construct. Both symbolic and adaptationist approaches to attachment thus share a concern for understanding the culturally relevant aspects of Strange Situation behavior; however, the symbolic approach prefers to examine attachment in light of meaning systems that go beyond functional adaptations to environmental circumstances.

Although the symbolic approach to culture has been well articulated by several researchers interested in the study of child development (Dunn, 1987; Garvey, 1992; P. J. Miller, 1982; Ochs & Schieffelin, 1984), it has not yet been applied to the study of attachment behavior. However, given its more cognitive focus, it may have a great deal to offer a theory of attachment that has emphasized the child's ability to process information and to construct patterns of meaning and social expectations on the basis of everyday interactions with significant adults. Moreover, a focus on symbolic meaning systems allows the cross-cultural investigator to examine directly the cultural constructs that inform behavior and its interpretation in culturally specific ways.

Finally, when one is considering cultural issues in attachment research, it is important to bear in mind that children grow up not within a single social or cultural context, but within a matrix of sociocultural contexts which are themselves both institutionally and socially constituted (Gergen, 1985; Shweder, 1990). Race, ethnicity, social class, religious affiliation, family composition, school environment, community makeup, and broader regional and national forces (e.g., the mass media) can all be viewed as contexts influencing the child. Moreover, these contexts are not simply the institutional structures that act as geophysical settings; they are also the tacit social and interactional norms of the individuals who exist within those settings, and whose behaviors and expectations both shape and are shaped by the institutional structures of which they are a part. From a symbolic perspective, it is in fact a misnomer to speak of "culture" at all, if by that term we imagine some one-to-one correspondence between "culture" and any one bounded geophysical or social entity. Rather, "culture" is best defined as an abstraction referring to the multiple meaningful contexts in which all individuals construct, and from which all individuals abstract, rule-governed understandings and behaviors (Gumperz & Hymes, 1986; Wartofsky, 1983).

CULTURAL ADAPTATIONISM: A CRITIQUE

There are several advantages to a cultural-adaptationist approach. First, it is relatively familiar to most psychologists through its historical association with evolutionary, ethological, and ecological thought. Second, it appeals to a model of scientific research that seeks to find lawful relationships and is accessible to objective measurement. Third, it gives serious consideration to the potential impact of different geophysical settings and specific caretaking practices on developmental outcomes. Finally, it focuses on the active role of the child in negotiating and influencing multiple interacting subsystems.

Unfortunately, cultural adaptationism in its fully elaborated form has also faced a variety of criticisms from both cultural anthropologists and cultural psychologists. Attachment researchers wishing to draw from this model should be aware of these criticisms in order to be able to select judiciously. First, anthropologists have questioned the tendency among many proponents of cultural adaptationism to talk about ecosystems as though they exist as isolable units; these researchers note that the modern world is characterized more by multiethnic contacts and the interpenetration of global and national systems than it is by bounded and isolable units (Cohen, 1978; Drummond, 1980; Smith, 1984). Moreover, any given individual is likely to claim membership in a number of ecosystems. For instance, the typical child in the United States today maintains multiple group memberships: Race, ethnicity, social class, religious affiliation, school, neighborhood, geographical region, family composition, and the mass media are just some of the common settings that children must learn to negotiate. The individual, then, must be viewed as an active organism existing within a matrix of sociocultural contexts or settings.

Second, an emphasis on functional interrelatedness among the different components of an ecosystem has been criticized for frequently confusing the genesis of practices with their current use (Geertz, 1973; Gould & Lewontin, 1979; Little, 1991). That is, a focus on functionalism has lent itself in the past to the telling of "just so" stories, in which the existence of a functional use for some characteristic (e.g., the giraffe's long neck enables it to eat the leaves of tall trees) is taken to be evidence concerning its genesis (i.e., the giraffe's long neck is considered an adaptive result of living in an environment full of tall trees). This leads to a spurious sense of causality, which undermines the explanatory power of functionalism. In fact, there is no provable causal connection between an environment of tall trees and the giraffe's long neck; instead, there is only a functional coexistence (see Gould & Lewontin, 1979). Similarly, in child development research the finding of two functionally interrelated practices (e.g., the use of open fires for cooking and heating, and caretakers' practice of carrying infants and toddlers on their backs) cannot be taken as evidence for a causal connection between these practices (e.g., "They carry the infants on their backs *so that* they won't be harmed by the open fires"). Moreover, the assumption that every cultural practice must have some functional utility has been questioned by several researchers. For instance, Sahlins (1976) suggests that the taboo in contemporary Western culture against eating dogs appears to be without functional utility, and is thus better understood from a symbolic perspective.

In addition, the identification of functional relationships does not permit us to formulate laws of co-occurrence that will generalize to other localities with similar environmental variables; in other words, it cannot be assumed that open fires and the practice of carrying infants and toddlers on one's back will necessarily co-occur in other cultural settings. Instead, multiple causes, multiple functions, and multiple outcomes appear to exist for any given phenomenon (Gollin, Stahl, & Morgan, 1989; Gould, 1980). Super and Harkness (1986) note, for instance, that interest in the "cultural ecology" school of cross-cultural child psychology has waned, in part because of a failure to find lawful relations between environmental variables and particular attitudes and behavior patterns.

Finally, the cognitive revolution within psychology has brought with it greater interest in the cognitive processing of social demands (e.g., Cole, 1983). This has paved the way for a more fluid, contextualized approach to social development, and has concomitantly allowed a shift of emphasis in the study of socialization from the general effects of specific child-rearing practices to the importance of everyday interactional routines as the matrix in which children learn the meaning of culturally appropriate behavior. Of increasing concern for many psychologists, then, is not so much finding lawful relationships among environmental variables and child-rearing practices, as identifying patterns of meaning that provide an interpretive framework for understanding the behavior of self and others, and that also serve to organize parent–infant interactions. In accordance with this, contemporary processual ecological approaches in anthropology and psychology (Boyd & Richerson, 1985; Tomasello, Kruger, & Ratner, 1993) emphasize both the dynamism of human ecological systems and the capacity of human symbolic powers to transform systems in unpredictable ways. This renders cognition a key variable in human ecology, culture, and evolution.

SYMBOLIC APPROACHES: A CRITIQUE

There are also several advantages of a symbolic approach to the study of culture. First, its emphasis on shared discourse and meaning systems rather than on personality variables makes it well suited to a

world in which interpenetration of systems, multiple cultural memberships, and systemic change are all increasingly common. According
to this view, attention shifts from the development of stable personality traits that are adaptive in a particular setting to the construction
of meanings that are relevant to given contexts. Just as children may
learn to be bilingual, so children may learn and integrate into a per-
sonally coherent whole the interactional strategies and symbolic meanings of different settings.

Second, a symbolic approach is more concerned with understanding the directive force of shared meaning systems in the lives of individuals (D'Andrade & Strauss, 1992; Harkness & Super, 1992) than
it is with finding lawful relationships among environmental variables,
caretaking practices, and behavioral outcomes. It may thus prove
useful to a cross-cultural enterprise that has encountered difficulty with
establishing the existence of such lawful relationships.

Third, symbolic approaches to the study of culture possess rich
possibilities for interdisciplinary dialogue, not only with cognitive
approaches within the field of psychology itself, but also with our sister
disciplines of anthropology and sociology. Within contemporary ecological anthropology, the importance of examining the role of symbolic
meaning systems is increasingly recognized (see Boyd & Richerson,
1985). The incorporation of a symbolic approach would allow attachment researchers to enter more fully into the theoretical debates and
paradigms that characterize the social sciences as a whole. Moreover,
given the complexity of individuals and the social structures that they
coconstitute, such an interdisciplinary approach to the study of child
development may be critical for future progress in the social sciences
(Gergen, 1985; J. G. Miller, 1994; Shweder, 1990).

Finally, it must be noted that attachment theory itself shows
multiple theoretical influences. In particular, its grounding in evolutionary theory and ethological research has made attachment theory
compatible with adaptationist approaches to culture. However, the
influence of information processing has also been profound (see in
particular Bowlby, 1980; Bretherton, 1985), thus rendering attachment theory equally amenable to symbolic approaches to culture.
Unfortunately, there has been a divergence in the field: Researchers
interested in the more clinical aspects of attachment (see Belsky &
Nezworski, 1988) have focused on the cognitive approach through
an examination of internal working models, whereas researchers interested in the more basic or experimental aspects of attachment (see
van IJzendoorn, 1990) have concentrated on investigating the adap-

tation of infants to different sociocultural niches. Significantly, however, the cognitive emphasis inherent in attachment theory makes it responsive not only to the clinical study of individual meanings, but to the cultural study of shared meanings as well, thus providing a unifying framework for these two divergent areas of inquiry within attachment research.

From this perspective, the study of meaning is a common enterprise, but the mental health meanings of individual differences in attachment can only be understood against the backdrop of the larger, cultural meanings given by different groups to desirable and undesirable child behavior. Just as our own cultural constructions have given us a normative framework within which to evaluate individual differences in attachment, so the study of other cultural belief systems may give us alternative normative frameworks within which to understand the culturally specific significance of individual differences in attachment behavior. The study of attachment, then, can adopt a common framework, but can differentiate between two distinct levels of inquiry within that framework: the level of shared or normative meaning that constitutes the realm of cross-cultural attachment research, and the level of idiographic meaning that comprises the domain of clinical attachment research (see Bowlby, 1980).

To turn to their disadvantages, symbolic approaches can be faulted for too often ignoring the ecology and social structures in which development occurs. However, as the work of Harkness and Super has demonstrated, a consideration of environmental setting is not necessarily antithetical to an analysis of symbolic meaning systems; it is at this point that the adaptationist and symbolic approaches may most fruitfully complement each other. In particular, Super and Harkness (1986; Harkness & Super, 1992) have developed a model for the cross-cultural study of the child that focuses on the "developmental niche." Briefly, the developmental niche is a theoretical framework for understanding the cultural regulation of the child's environment. It consists of three components: the physical and social settings in which the child lives; the customs of child care and child rearing; and the psychology of the caretakers, including their cultural meaning systems or "parental ethnotheories," which are assigned a leading role in this framework. Super and Harkness argue that these three subsystems interact with one another, and that together they provide a framework for the individual's developmental experience, as well as for cultural variation in that experience.

Second, some researchers may object to the use of a symbolic approach to the cross-cultural study of attachment, on the grounds that it lacks rigor. There are two levels at which this criticism may occur. The extent to which symbolic approaches focus on culturally constituted meaning systems rather than the discovery of universal laws may be considered by some as not in keeping with a true scientific spirit, and the use of qualitative data may be viewed as empirically nonrigorous. However, the context-specific description of particular settings has been part of developmental research ever since naturalistic observation became a common and valued tool (see Barker & Gump, 1964; Bronfenbrenner, 1977). In addition, Tomasello et al. (1993) offer evidence that endorsement of the importance of symbolic meaning systems in child development may coexist coherently with the view that universal laws operating within biological evolution have led to the capacity for culture and its diversity. Finally, as researchers have demonstrated (Harwood, 1992; J. G. Miller, 1984; J. G. Miller, Bersoff, & Harwood, 1990), conventional empirical standards of methodological rigor need not be compromised through taking a more qualitative approach to the understanding of different cultural meaning systems.

Third, some researchers may object to the relativistic stance of a symbolic approach, noting that the existence of cultural differences in mothers' perceptions of attachment behavior does not mean that the secure base system works differently across cultures (L. A. Sroufe, personal communication, 1992). This is certainly true, and in response a distinction must be made between basic human mechanisms that evidence suggests are universal, particularly in infancy, and the cultural constructs that human beings have built in an attempt to understand those mechanisms. For instance, the human reproductive system works identically across cultures; nonetheless, the cultural constructs people have created regarding the sexual and marital relationships in which human reproduction occurs show vast cross-cultural variation. Similarly, evidence suggests that it may be a human universal in later infancy for the subsystems of affiliation, wariness, exploration, and attachment to work together in coherent and recognizable patterns. It may even be that a sense of safety and emotional warmth underlie patterns of attachment behavior that are deemed desirable across a majority of cultures. However, these issues are separate from the cultural construct of security that we have created in U.S. psychology on the basis of these mechanisms. In particular, the concept of inner security, with its emphasis on the importance of self-sufficiency and inner resourcefulness for the autonomous, bounded individual, who is nonetheless capable of existing harmoniously and finding satisfaction in relationships with other autonomous, bounded individuals, is an ideal peculiar to dominant U.S. culture—a culturally constructed developmental endpoint that is not shared by much of the rest of the world. The cultural constructs built on the basic human mechanisms are what provide the cross-cultural variations in meaning systems of interest to a symbolic approach.

Finally, some psychologists have criticized symbolic approaches for seeming to assume that all members of a given sociocultural group will maintain identical meaning systems, thus ignoring or discounting within-group variability (e.g., Turiel, 1983). As J. G. Miller (1994) notes, however, a cultural perspective leads to the expectation of both individual differences and contextual variations in behavior. We explore this issue more fully in Chapter Six.

CONCLUSION

In summary, cross-cultural research on attachment has tended to draw upon an adaptationist model for understanding the role of culture. We believe that a symbolic approach may also prove fruitful in our attempts to understand the cultural shaping of attachment, by allowing us to explore the meanings given to various Strange Situation behaviors by members of different sociocultural groups. In addition, by gaining greater insight into some of the cultural constructs that shape our understanding of desirable and undesirable socialization goals, we can better evaluate the culturally relevant meaning of individual differences in attachment behavior.

CHAPTER THREE

Studying Culture and Attachment: A Symbolic Approach

◆

In this chapter, we provide an overview of the method and results used in two studies examining perceptions of attachment behavior among Anglo and Puerto Rican mothers. As other researchers have noted (Denzin & Lincoln, 1994; J. G. Miller, 1994), there is no bounded set of methodologies associated with cultural psychology. Instead, reflecting the interdisciplinary nature of the field, cultural psychology studies tend to employ a variety of strategies (e.g., quantitative and interpretive, comparative and noncomparative). The studies under discussion in this book combine a symbolic approach (i.e., an interest in the study of symbolic meaning systems) with both quantitative and interpretive methodologies, in order to examine sociocultural differences in the meanings given to desirable and undesirable attachment behavior among four groups of mothers: middle- and working-class mainland Anglo, and middle- and working-class island Puerto Rican.[1]

We also examine those meanings using quantitative methods and conventional standards of empirical rigor in this chapter. For instance, if symbolic meaning systems constitute, to some extent, shared discourse, then it should be possible to study their "shared" aspect em-

---

[1]"Middle-class" mothers were actually drawn from the top two strata of Hollingshead's (1975) socioeconomic scaling instrument (major and minor business, professional, and technical workers); "working-class" mothers were actually drawn from Hollingshead's lowest two strata (semiskilled and unskilled workers). We are using the terms "middle-class" and working-class" for the sake of brevity.

pirically, that is, what is shared and to what extent? In Chapters Four through Six, we examine those meanings using a more interpretive methodology (i.e., a methodology grounded in the traditions of qualitative discourse analysis). In other words, as shared "discourse," we attempt to explicate some of the rich levels of meaning inherent in the content of mothers' responses.

Finally, a word must be said regarding group commonality and within-group variability. We have argued that, from a symbolic perspective, culture is not an isolable entity but a process of finding and negotiating shared meaning between social interactants. If this is true, then the four sociocultural units we have constructed for the purpose of this study ("middle-" and "working-class" "Anglo" and "Puerto Rican" mothers) are to some extent arbitrary; we could just as easily have chosen to compare how meaning is negotiated in a classroom of U.S. sixth-graders in suburban Chicago versus how it is negotiated in an inner-city classroom in the same city. On the other hand, if culture can be understood as shared meaning systems, then it should be possible to find a level at which meaning is shared by mothers from a common national background, as well as by mothers from a particular socioeconomic background. Because most attachment research has focused on national and socioeconomic group differences, we have thus chosen to focus on these differences in this research as well. However, it is important to keep in mind that both within-group commonality and within-group variability exist for each of our four sociocultural groups, and we will examine both in later chapters.

STUDY 1: INDIGENOUS PERCEPTIONS OF BEHAVIOR

The purpose of Study 1 was to examine indigenous perceptions of adult socialization goals, child behavior, and desirable and undesirable attachment behavior among Anglo and Puerto Rican mothers. We expected that such an undertaking would enable us to gain greater insight into some of the ways in which cultural meaning systems shape mothers' views regarding desirable and undesirable adult and child socialization outcomes. In addition, we were interested in examining the possible influence of these larger socialization goals on mothers' interpretations of individual differences in attachment behavior. Finally, we hoped to increase our understanding of the specific meaning systems endorsed by Anglo and Puerto Rican mothers across a range of socioeconomic backgrounds.

Study Participants

Four groups consisting of 20 mothers each participated in Study 1. All mothers were at least 20 years of age, and had a toddler aged 12–24 months—the age during which the Strange Situation is normally used to assess attachment behavior (Ainsworth & Wittig, 1969). There were no group differences in the age of each mother's Strange Situation-age child (mean = 17.4 months), and gender distribution was equal across the four groups. The Anglo mothers were drawn from New Haven County in Connecticut, were white mothers of non-Hispanic European ancestry who had been born and educated in the United States, and spoke English as their first language. The Puerto Rican mothers were drawn from the San Juan–Caguas and Ponce areas, had lived in Puerto Rico their entire lives, and spoke Spanish as their first language.

The Hollingshead (1975) four-factor scale was used to determine socioeconomic status when two employed adults were present in the household; when the household contained one or no wage earners, socioeconomic status was ascertained for the head of household according to Hollingshead's two-factor scale. The measure constructed by Hollingshead is a scaling instrument that yields discrete socioeconomic status groups based on education and occupational prestige.

New Haven, Connecticut

Connecticut is the third smallest U.S. state in area, measuring roughly 90 miles long and 75 miles wide. With Massachusetts and Rhode Island to the north and east, Connecticut is part of New England as well as one of the original 13 colonies, and has a strong and proud Yankee tradition. In addition, bordered on the south by Long Island Sound and on the west by New York, Connecticut serves not only as a residential area for upscale New Yorkers seeking a suburban setting, but also as a migration point for a variety of ethnic groups aspiring to life outside New York City.

In the south central section of Connecticut, the city of New Haven marks the eastern terminus of the metropolitan commuter train line into Manhattan. With New York City 80 miles to the southwest and Boston 140 miles to the northeast, New Haven lies squarely on the highly traveled "Northeast corridor" that runs from Washington, D.C., to Boston. The state capital of Hartford (also considered to be on the corridor) is about 45 miles north.

The city of New Haven is Connecticut's third largest, with 130,474 residents within the city limits in 1990. Surrounding the city of New Haven proper are its 28 suburban towns, covering approximately 482 square miles; the city and the towns together make up New Haven County. Total population for Connecticut in 1990 was 3,287,116.[2] Of these, 804,214 people, or roughly 25% of the state's population, lived in New Haven County, making it one of the most populous of Connecticut's eight counties.

New Haven, like Connecticut as a whole, is a study in contrasts. The state itself is one of the wealthiest in the United States, with a median family income in 1989 of $49,199 (the national median family income was $35,225); New Haven County, with a median family income of $46,058, was the 12th richest in the country in the 1990 census. On the other hand, three major Connecticut cities (Hartford, New Haven, and Bridgeport) all rank among the 15 worst metropolitan areas in the United States in terms of discrepancy between city and suburban income. In particular, the 28 towns that surround New Haven had a median family income of $53,886 in 1989, whereas in New Haven itself the median family income was just $31,163. In 1990, 23% of New Haven residents lived in poverty (defined that year by the federal government as an income of $12,674 for a family of four), while only 4% of county suburban residents did.

New Haven County presents a similar study in ethnic contrasts. For instance, nearly 22% of area residents identified themselves in the 1990 census as Italian-American, and numerous other white ethnic groups are also well represented both inside and outside the city. Yet the urban–suburban disparity in New Haven County is stark when racial differences are considered: No fewer than 93% of suburban residents in the 1990 census were white; in contrast, whites accounted for only 49% of the city's residents. In the 1980s, the Hispanic population throughout the country grew by 53%; however, Spanish-speaking minorities (primarily Puerto Rican) grew by nearly 80% in New Haven, accounting in 1990 for 13.2% of the city's population but only 2.2% of the suburban population.

[2]All U.S., Connecticut, and Puerto Rican census information in this chapter is drawn from U.S. Bureau of the Census (1990).

Middle-Class Anglo Mothers

Accordingly, only 45% of the middle-class Anglo mothers in this study lived within the city of New Haven, while 55% resided in the surrounding suburbs (30% in Hamden, a comfortable middle-class suburb just north of the city limits). All but one were affiliated either through their own or their husbands' occupations with Yale University or Yale–New Haven Hospital; these two institutions are the county's two largest employers, together employing over 15,000 people.

The middle-class Anglo mothers in our sample were contacted through advertisements in the *Yale Weekly Bulletin & Calendar*, a newsletter distributed throughout the university and hospital communities. Nine of the middle-class Anglo mothers were affiliated with Yale as staff members or administrators; four were either graduate students, faculty members, or wives of faculty or graduate students; two were professionally employed alumnae living in the area; and four were other professionals serving within the university system (e.g., as a nurse/midwife or recreation therapist at one of the medical facilities). The average Hollingshead occupational prestige score was 57.4, or that of a professional. All of the middle-class Anglo mothers were married, and most were college-educated and worked outside the home (see Table 1). In summary, the middle-class Anglo mothers in this study were a largely professional, highly educated group of women living in an area of the United States where the disparity between the "haves" and the "have-nots" is particularly stark.

Working-Class Anglo Mothers

Forty percent of the working-class Anglo mothers who participated in our study lived in East Haven, a largely working-class community (pop. 26,144, 1990 census) located immediately to New Haven's east, where the presence of industry has lowered the property values in adjacent neighborhoods. East Haven's median family income in 1989 was $42,797, compared to $53,886 in the suburban area as a whole. The remaining 60% lived in other, similarly less privileged New Haven suburbs.

The working-class Anglo mothers were contacted through Women, Infants, and Children (WIC) programs within the city of New Haven. Many of the working-class mothers reached these services via the city and county bus systems, while others arranged for neighbors or relatives to drive them; privately owned transportation was rare.

TABLE 1. Demographic Characteristics, Middle-Class Mothers, Study 1

Characteristic	Anglo	Puerto Rican
Target child's age (months)	17.0	17.7
Mother's age	32.0	29.1*
Mother's education (years)	16.5	15.5*
% mothers employed	85.0	80.0
% working full-time	45.0	60.0
No. of hours worked per week	26.7	27.3
% married	100.0	80.0
Total no. of children	1.5	1.6
Household size (no. of people)	3.6	3.8
Father's education	17.0	15.8
Hollingshead score	57.4	53.1

Note. $n = 20$ in each group.
*$p < .05$.

The working-class Anglo mothers in our sample were on average younger and less educated than the middle-class group (see Table 2). Just over half were unmarried, only one-quarter worked outside the home, and 65% were on welfare (Aid to Families with Dependent Children, or AFDC). Thirty percent of the mothers were single and living in households in which no employed adult was present; 45% were married with at least one employed adult in the house; the remaining 25% were single but living with relatives, at least one of whom was employed. The average Hollingshead occupational prestige score among the working-class Anglo mothers was 24.9, or that of a semi-skilled laborer. Among the mothers in wage-earning households, 10 had husbands or partners in traditional blue-collar occupations (e.g., manufacturing, auto repair, construction), and four were themselves employed in service industries (e.g., as a cashier, waitress, or clerical worker). Only one of the working-class Anglo mothers was affiliated with Yale University, through her job as a clerical assistant.

Puerto Rico

Lying between the Atlantic Ocean and the Caribbean Sea, Puerto Rico is the easternmost and smallest of the Greater Antilles islands. The annual temperature across the island averages 77°F. One hundred ten miles long and 35 miles wide, Puerto Rico has a central mountain range running most of its length, which effectively divides the island into

TABLE 2. Demographic Characteristics, Working-Class Mothers, Study 1

Characteristic	Anglo	Puerto Rican
Target child's age (months)	17.5	17.5
Mother's age	24.7	25.3
Mother's education (years)	11.4	10.2
% mothers employed	25.0	25.0
% working full-time	15.0	15.0
No. of hours worked per week	8.4	7.3
% married	45.0	50.0
Total no. of children	1.5	1.8
Household size (no. of people)	3.6	3.9
Father's education	11.5	10.8
Hollingshead score	24.9	19.4
% on AFDC (welfare)	65.0	65.0

Note. n = 20 in each group.

northern and southern coastal regions. The northern coast, facing the Atlantic Ocean, is wetter and greener than the southern coast, and also contains most of the island's major metropolitan areas. The southern coast faces the Caribbean Sea and has one principal city, Ponce. A major highway runs from north to south across the central mountain region, connecting San Juan with Ponce, about an hour's drive away.

A Brief History

Columbus first encountered Puerto Rico in 1493 on his second voyage to the New World, and in 1508, Ponce de León established the first Spanish settlement on the island in the area that was to become known as San Juan. The native population of Taino Indians did not long survive the Spanish conquest; most of the Tainos were either killed or had died of disease by the mid-16th century, and the remaining few were absorbed into the conquering population. The island's metal deposits were also exhausted by the mid-16th century, and thus Puerto Rico became less attractive to its early colonizers. For nearly 200 years thereafter, the island was used chiefly as a port and as a military bastion for the defense of Spanish vessels on their way to the Spanish-American mainland. Spain began to concern itself with making Puerto Rico a productive colony only at the beginning of the 19th century, when the Spanish Empire's disintegration made the island a refuge for Spanish families fleeing from newly independent mainland colonies.

As a result of attendant social and economic changes, Puerto Rican society was transformed during the 19th century from a basically smallholding, peasant subsistence economy to a predominantly seignorial economy of moderate-sized haciendas producing cash crops for export (primarily sugar cane, tobacco, and coffee). In 1898, Spain ceded Puerto Rico to the United States following the Spanish-American War, and Puerto Ricans were granted U.S. citizenship status in 1917. Because sugar was one of the few products that the mainland United States did not produce abundantly, Puerto Rico filled a crucial economic need; within 25 years of the island's becoming a U.S. possession, sugar cane had become the primary cash crop, accounting for 66% of total exports in 1920. When the island's sugar industry went into decline with the global depression of the 1930s, the results were rampant unemployment, poverty, and political ferment (Bethell, 1986; Carr, 1984; Centro de Estudios Puertorriqueños, 1979).

Since World War II, Puerto Rico has carved out a unique and not uncontroversial political relationship with the United States. In 1948, the U.S. Congress authorized the direct election of the governor of Puerto Rico by its people—an election that resulted in the resounding victory of the Partido Popular Democrático (PPD). The PPD, under the leadership of Luis Muñoz Marín, became the driving force of Puerto Rico's development in the decades following World War II. Essentially, the PPD took a moderate, populist, but pragmatic stance toward independence from the United States, seeking a middle ground between the pro-statehood and *independentista* groups.

By the end of World War II, the pro-statehood movement had become identified in Puerto Rico with the largely absentee-owned corporate interests that had dominated the sugar economy, and was thus a target of popular discontent; the *independentistas*, on the other hand, fought an uphill battle with the economic reality that Puerto Rico had benefited greatly from the New Deal aid and reconstruction programs legislated in the 1930s. The PPD inherited from its political forerunners a belief that the issue of Puerto Rico's legal status with the United States was basically irrelevant to the larger task of bettering the condition of the average laborer. As Bethell (1990, p. 582) notes, "pragmatism was stronger than independentism in the ideological armory of the PPD, which was closer to the New Dealism of Roosevelt" than it was to either nationalism or socialism.

Following his election in 1948, Muñoz Marín began to move toward the political compromise that would become known in English as the Commonwealth of Puerto Rico and in Spanish as the Estado Libre Asociado. A constitution was ratified in 1952 providing for internal self-government; this "solved" the colonial political dilemma, but allowed federal administrative and military agencies to continue to operate fully on the island, thus leaving in place the existing infrastructure (which, it was hoped, would preserve the conditions for economic progress). Since 1952, the PPD and the pro-statehood party have become increasingly balanced politically, setting the stage for gridlock between the two parties and a consequential maintenance of the original commonwealth solution (Bethell, 1990).

In terms of social and economic change, the years of commonwealth status have seen a rapid industrialization of Puerto Rico. By 1980, only 4% of the island's net income came from agriculture, compared to over 31% in 1940. Concomitant to this industrialization has been a massive migration: Almost half (44%) of Puerto Rico's total population of 6,249,791 now lives on the mainland United States. This migration has been accompanied by relatively rapid depopulation of the rural central mountain region and by relatively rapid growth of the major metropolitan areas, particularly San Juan. By 1990, 56% of Puerto Rico's 3.5 million inhabitants— nearly 2 million people—resided in the San Juan–Caguas metropolitan area, and nearly 1.7 million in the greater San Juan area; over 458,000 lived in the city of San Juan itself. Ponce, the island's second largest metropolitan area outside San Juan, contained 232,947 residents in 1990.

Culturally, a major factor in favor of commonwealth status as opposed to statehood has been a concern for the preservation of Puerto Rican identity. Military service in the U.S. armed forces, return migration from the United States, U.S. business in Puerto Rico, and the mass media have all been significant "Americanizing" influences on the island. Prior to Puerto Rico's first popular gubernatorial election in 1948, English was the primary language in public schools. Following the election of Muñoz Marín, instruction in Spanish was set at all levels of public education, with English taught as a compulsory second language. The perpetuation of Puerto Rican identity remains a strong concern on the island, and is closely tied to the maintenance of Spanish as a first language for all Puerto Rican residents.

Economically, Puerto Rico continues to be substantially poorer than the mainland United States. In 1989, the median family income for the island as a whole was $9,988, and 58.9% of the population was living below the federally determined poverty line.

Middle-Class Puerto Rican Mothers

The middle-class Puerto Rican mothers in our sample were drawn from the San Juan–Caguas–Bayamon–Carolina metropolitan area in the northeastern quarter of the island, and from Ponce, the southern coast's major city and Puerto Rico's second largest metropolitan area. In 1990, as noted above, over one-half (1,994,002) of Puerto Rico's island population of 3,522,037 resided in the San Juan area; another 232,947 lived in Ponce. As Puerto Rico's capital, San Juan contains the island's principal governmental, cultural, and educational institutions, including the main campus of the University of Puerto Rico, which is located in the San Juan suburb of Río Piedras. The University of Puerto Rico also maintains a campus in Ponce.

Forty percent of the 20 middle-class Puerto Rican mothers who participated in Study 1 lived in the university town of Río Piedras; 45% resided in other San Juan suburban towns; and 15% lived in Ponce. Eighteen of the mothers were affiliated with the University of Puerto Rico at Río Piedras (including two of the Ponce mothers), 15 as alumni and 3 as current students.

Culturally, eliciting subject participation in Puerto Rico requires face-to-face contact and personal invitation. In order to observe the cultural norms and also achieve a range of mothers in the final sample, 20 different graduate students in education classes at the Río Piedras campus were each asked to find two mothers (one middle- and one working-class) who met sampling criteria with regard to age of target child, socioeconomic status, Puerto Rican ethnic identity, and lifelong residence on the island. The resultant sample of 40 mothers did not know one another, worked in different settings, and lived in a variety of neighborhoods throughout the metropolitan San Juan and Ponce areas.

All but five of the middle-class Puerto Rican mothers had a college degree or higher, and three of these five were in their final years of undergraduate study. Eighty percent were married, two were unmarried but living with the fathers of their children, and two were divorced; one of the divorced women had moved back into her family of origin's home.

Eighty percent of the middle-class Puerto Rican mothers worked outside the home, mostly as professionals (six teachers and four health professionals), or at the managerial level in government, business, and educational settings. Among the four women who did not work outside the home, three had husbands in professional or managerial positions, and the fourth mother was divorced and living with her family of origin. The average Hollingshead occupational prestige score was 53.1, or that of a professional.

As can be seen in Table 1, of the 11 demographic variables examined in Study 1, the middle-class Puerto Rican mothers differed from the middle-class Anglo mothers on just two: They were younger, and had on average 1 year less of higher education. The two groups did not differ in terms of three indices of maternal employment status (percentage employed outside home, percentage working full-time, and number of hours worked per week), marital status, total number of children, household size, father's education, or Hollingshead occupational prestige score. However, middle-class Puerto Rican mothers were less likely than middle-class Anglo mothers to be living in a household consisting of a husband, wife, and children (respective means = 75% as compared to 100%). Instead, two of the Puerto Rican mothers were unmarried but living with the fathers of their children; two were divorced (one of these women, as noted, had moved back into her family of origin's home); and one was married, but she and her husband had relatives living with them.

In summary, despite Puerto Rico's substantial poverty, the middle-class mothers in our sample maintained a comfortable lifestyle, were employed at a professional or managerial level, and were relatively well educated (nationally, only 20.3% of U.S. citizens had college degrees or higher in the 1990 census, compared to 75% of our middle-class Puerto Rican sample and 85% of our middle-class Anglo mothers). Given the additional facts that both the Anglo and the Puerto Rican middle-class mothers were affiliated with university communities, lived in suburban neighborhoods surrounding major metropolitan areas, and enjoyed relatively privileged lives in the context of a fair amount of poverty, it would appear that these mothers constituted adequate comparison groups. Finally, although none of our Puerto Rican mothers had ever lived on the mainland United States, Puerto Rico's commonwealth status renders U.S. influence omnipresent, particularly among the educated, metropolitan middle classes. One could reasonably speculate that our middle-class Puerto Rican mothers were actually relatively "Americanized" compared to other mothers on the island, thus providing a conservative test for cultural differences.

Working-Class Puerto Rican Mothers

Although working-class Anglo mothers had been contacted without incident through WIC programs in New Haven, cultural norms regarding personal contact and dignity made it difficult in Puerto Rico to work through impersonal government agencies such as WIC programs. Working-class Puerto Rican mothers were therefore contacted directly in federally subsidized housing complexes in the San Juan and Ponce areas by graduate students in education classes at the Río Piedras campus.

In highly urbanized San Juan, these housing complexes tended to be larger, more impersonal, and more dangerous than they were in the smaller city of Ponce, and thus the majority (70%) of our working-class Puerto Rican mothers resided in the Ponce area, while the remaining 30% lived in San Juan. Moreover, it was felt that the low-income housing areas in Ponce tended to approximate more closely the poorer neighborhoods of suburban New Haven County than did the inner-city slums of San Juan. However, in order to insure that working-class San Juan and Ponce mothers were culturally similar, t tests were performed comparing these two groups on all study results.

The working-class Puerto Rican mothers, like their Anglo counterparts, were on average younger and less educated than the middle-class mothers (see Table 2). Only 25% of them worked outside the home, half were unmarried, and 65% were on welfare (AFDC). Thirty percent were single, unemployed mothers; 45% were married and living in a household with at least one employed adult present; the remaining 25% were unemployed, living with unemployed relatives. The average Hollingshead score was 19.4, on the boundary in Hollingshead's categories between skilled and unskilled labor. Among the mothers living in wage-earning households, three had husbands employed in traditional blue-collar occupations; one husband worked as an agricultural laborer; and five mothers were themselves employed in service industries (e.g., as a cashier, hairdresser, or clerical worker).

As can be seen in Table 2, the working-class Puerto Rican mothers did not differ from the working-class Anglo mothers on any of 12 demographic variables. The two groups did not differ in terms of mothers' age or education, three indices of maternal employment status (percentage employed outside home, percentage working full-time, and number of hours worked per week), marital status, total number of children, household size, father's education, Hollingshead occupational prestige score, or welfare status. In addition, the composition of the households that mothers lived in (i.e., whether spouses, parents, or other relatives lived with them) did not differ.

Procedures Used

Study 1 consisted of open-ended, individually administered interviews conducted by ethnically matched, trained interviewers in subjects' homes. The interviews were tape-recorded and transcribed verbatim for further analysis. The Spanish version of the interview protocol was obtained through standard back-translation techniques. Each interview took about 45 minutes to an hour to complete.

Long-Term Socialization Goals

In order to obtain indigenous conceptualizations of desirable and undesirable social behavior, mothers were asked four open-ended questions. The first two questions probed for values concerning long-term socialization goals:

1. "Most mothers, when they have a child, have some idea about what sorts of qualities they would like their children to possess—what kind of person they would like their children to grow up to be. When you think about your children, what sorts of qualities would you like them to possess as they grow older?"

2. "Again, most mothers have some idea about what sorts of qualities they would really *not* like ther children to possess. When you think about your children, what sorts of qualities would you *not* want them to possess as they grow older?"

Desirable and Undesirable Child Behavior

In order to obtain a fuller picture of culturally valued behavior, the next two questions probed for desirable and undesirable toddler behavior in relation to these long-term socialization goals:

3. "You have just told me some of the qualities that you would like your children to possess. Now I want you to think about a child you know between the ages of 1 and 2 who has at least the beginnings of some of those qualities. It can be either your own child or another child you know. Of course, all children have both good and bad qualities, but right now think just about that child's good qualities. Now I'd like you to describe that child's personality, or at least the 'good' side of that child's personality."

4. "You told me before about some of the qualities that you would *not* like your children to possess. Now I want you to think about a child you know between the ages of 1 and 2 who has at least the beginnings of some of those qualities. It can be either your own child or another child you know. Of course, all children have both good and bad qualities, but right now think just about that child's bad qualities. Now I'd like you to describe that child's personality, or at least the 'bad' side of that child's personality."

It was anticipated that the responses to questions 1 and 2 would provide information concerning abstract, idealized adult qualities, and that questions 3 and 4 would elicit more contextualized descriptions. We felt that examination of the coherence between perceptions of desirable child behavior and of ideal adult endpoints should yield a rich picture of mothers' indigenous conceptualizations of desirable and undesirable toddler behavior in relation to long-term socialization goals.

Desirable and Undesirable Attachment Behavior

The Strange Situation was chosen as the vehicle for investigating mothers' perceptions of attachment behavior because it is both standardized and widely used. Following the four open-ended probes, indigenous concepts of Strange Situation behavior were elicited from the mothers with questions designed to replicate the three main phases (preseparation, separation, and reunion) of the Strange Situation. A drawing of the setting was supplied on the basis of the Strange Situation literature (Ainsworth et al., 1978) in order to facilitate mothers' visualization of the task (see Figure 1). Specifically, mothers were first asked to imagine how the desirable toddler they had described in question 3 would behave in a setting (the waiting room of a doctor's office) that simulated the primary features of the Strange Situation:

5a. "Now I'd like you to think about the boy/girl you described to me earlier—the one who you feel possesses qualities that are really good for a child between the ages of 1 and 2 to possess. First, we need to call this child by a name. You can use either the child's real name, or any other name you would like. Okay, now we're going to think about [name] in a specific situation, and imagine what he/she would do in that situation. [Show picture of Strange Situation.] Here's a

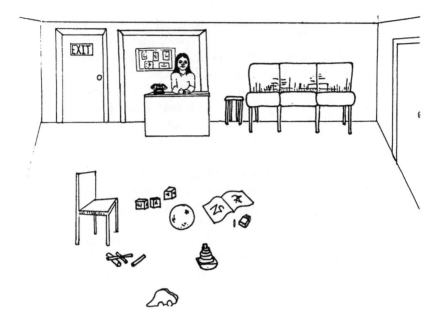

FIGURE 1. The drawing of the Strange Situation setting that was shown to mothers in our research.

drawing of the waiting room of a doctor's office. [Describe room, point out doors, couch, toys, and receptionist.] First, be sure to picture [name] as being between 1 and 2 years old. [Name] has just come into the waiting room with his/her mother. The mother sits down on the couch. What does [name] do?"

5b. "Now let's imagine that the doctor asks to see the mother briefly. Let's imagine that the mother knows it will only take a minute and feels comfortable leaving the child very briefly in the waiting room with the receptionist, whom the mother knows slightly. The child does not know the receptionist. The mother says, 'Goodbye, [name], I'll be right back,' and leaves the room. What does [name] do?"

5c. "Now let's imagine that the mother returns to the waiting room after having been gone a couple of minutes. She says, 'Hi, [name].' What does [name] do?"

These questions were then repeated (as questions 6a, 6b, and 6c) for the undesirable toddler mothers had described in question 4. If mothers paused more than 15 seconds before beginning to answer the questions, they were prompted with two general questions designed to be as nonleading as possible: "Where in the room would [name] be? What would he/she be doing?" The majority of mothers did not require any prompting.

Creation of Coding Categories

In order to identify culturally relevant dimensions of toddler behavior, we analyzed subjects' responses to questions 1 through 4 at the level of individual word and phrase descriptors. For instance, "that they not pick up vices and they behave well" counted as two phrase descriptors, whereas "honest and decent and treat people with respect" counted as two word descriptors and one phrase descriptor.

Individual word and phrase descriptors were coded into six mutually exclusive categories. We chose to call the first of these categories Self-Maximization; it included all responses generated by mothers indicating concern that a child become self-confident and independent, and develop his or her talents and abilities as an individual. (In the following examples and in all other maternal responses quoted in this book, the numbers are the code numbers mothers were assigned in the course of our research.)

> #153: I would like to make sure that she feels secure enough to just try lots of different things and to be creative in her ways of expression—not to fall into standard patterns. I don't want her to be a coloring-book child. I want her to have paints and crayons that she does whatever she wants with. And—but I guess part of that still relates to fear—being afraid of expressing her own self. I just want her to feel free.

> #148: I don't really want them to limit themselves. I want them to feel like the world is their oyster, and it's there for them. I don't want them to set limitations, basically. . . . I always want them to believe that no matter what it is that they can try hard enough— and if they don't make it, at least they've felt like they've given it 100%. That's very important. I don't ever want them to look back and say "I should have" or "I might have." I want them to be the best that they can be, whatever that is for them.

The second category, Self-Control, contained all responses indicating concern that a child learn to curb negative impulses toward greed, egocentrism, and aggression—or, put positively, to learn to share, accept limits, and cope with frustration:

> #156: He's a really intense child and he'll always be that way. It's just his—it's just the way he's wired. And so, umm, just not being a hothead, blow up easy about things, have a tantrum—to be more—being able to cool off and think about things and be a little more rational. . . . The kid will not share. Any toy my son picks up he rips it out of his hands, whether it's his toy or my son's.

> #151: He's incredibly, umm, easily frustrated, and every little thing sort of sets him off. Well, he used to bang his head. He'd get so frustrated about something, you know, that he'd bang his— he just couldn't handle it. He just couldn't cope with, like, not being able to put a puzzle piece in. He'd sort of throw the puzzle piece across the floor, throw himself on the floor, and bang his head.

The third category, Lovingness, contained all responses indicating concern that a child be friendly, emotionally warm, and able to maintain close affective bonds with others:

> #02: [She's] very [affectionate], very friendly. No matter where I go with her—to the market, to the movies, or to eat at a restaurant—she gets everyone's attention, she touches everyone's heart. That is when I notice how loving she is. She touches people when she gets close to them; immediately she breaks that person's heart, because that person, well, immediately gives her attention, carries her, or attempts to kiss her, touch her, because she is so [affectionate].

> #156: I'll always remember—this little boy walking around with his stuffed animals, kissing them and hugging them and just being a really kind of a sweet, sweet kid.

The fourth category, Decency, contained all responses indicating concern that a child grow up to meet basic societal standards of integrity, such as being a hard-working, responsible, and honest person who does not use drugs:

> #164: I hope he doesn't become a troublemaker. And I hope he doesn't get into drugs, because I don't think I could take it. And I've seen little kids already that learned to lie. And I can't stand it. That's one thing that had better stop before it starts. And stealing.

#167: Well, they watch their father not working and stuff, so that's why my brother takes them [to work with him]: It shows them responsibility to work and stuff, which their father never did. . . . Be working instead of sitting around like a bum all the time. Can't raise a family or support yourself being a bum.

The fifth category, Proper Demeanor, contained all responses indicating concern that a child be well mannered, well behaved, cooperative, and accepted by the larger community, and that parents likewise perform their parental duties appropriately:

#03: The little girl is [obedient]; even though she is young, [she respects] her mother and things like that. Well, [she is obedient] because every time the mother tells her to come and sit down, she comes, eats her food and everything. Mine, at least up to now, doesn't eat food or sit down [when I tell her], or anything like that. Well, give respect to elders and to the people around her, do this just the same in school as at home.

#38: All the things that are bad manners—like crying for no apparent reason, saying bad words, disrespect toward their elders—these tend to be very charming at [a young] age. . . . [But later] it begins to be bothersome, and then he is rejected: "Take this child, I can't take him any more. Look, he did this ill-mannered thing to me, he did this to me, he did that to me.". . . Perhaps that is one of the reasons I would not like it—because he would end up feeling rejected, including feeling others' harsh looks because he is like that. Nobody wants to take care of [a poorly brought-up child]; nobody wants to be with him.

The final category, Miscellaneous, contained all content responses that could not be coded in the first five categories (e.g., "She's not a big television watcher," "cute," "I wouldn't like him to grow up to be a conservative Republican"). It must be emphasized that fewer than 5% of mothers' responses across all groups were coded as Miscellaneous, attesting to the broadly encompassing character of the five content categories. In addition to these categories, most interviews contained remarks that were not coded at all because they were considered vague (e.g., "He's terrific"), extraneous (e.g., "I don't know that many children, but I know some with bad qualities"), contextual (e.g., "She's 5, I'd say"), or of a commentary nature ("The little one, she's just picking up from her brother").

Reliability in coding mothers' open-ended conceptualizations of desirable and undesirable social behavior was calculated between the first author (Harwood) and one independent judge on 50% of the sample. Overall agreement reached a satisfactory level of .83 (Cohen's kappa; range = .81–.86).

Analysis of Category Usage

The analysis of possible differences in category use was complicated by the fact that although middle-class Anglo and Puerto Rican mothers gave a similar number of responses to study questions (respective means = 79 and 76), both these groups gave more responses than did the working-class Anglo mothers (mean = 63), who in turn differed from the working-class Puerto Rican mothers (mean = 40 responses). This conclusion is based on an analysis of variance (ANOVA) using post hoc Tukey tests for differences among means ($p < .05$). Because of this difference in verbal fluency, analyses involving differences in category use employed percentages rather than frequencies. In addition, arc–sine transformations appropriate for the use of proportional data were performed on all subsequent analyses involving percentages.

San Juan versus Ponce Mothers

Because of the possible differences in background between the working-class San Juan and Ponce mothers in Puerto Rico, an examination was undertaken to demonstrate their comparability for the purposes of this study. In particular, t tests were performed comparing San Juan and Ponce mothers on all study results. The results indicated that working-class San Juan and Ponce mothers differed on only 2 of 31 variables, and the categories involved (Lovingness, and Expresses Anger in the Strange Situation) were not ones that reflected cultural differences in the larger analysis. As for the middle-class mothers, all but three of them lived in San Juan, and two of the exceptions had studied in San Juan. In both groups, therefore, combining mothers from the two geographic areas seemed reasonable and neutral with regard to the overall study results.

Open-Ended Conceptualizations

To compare subjects' responses to the four open-ended questions, a $4 \times 4 \times 6$ (group × question × category type) ANOVA was performed on the relative percentages of subjects' descriptors that could be coded into each of the categories. This ANOVA yielded significant main effects for group, $F(3, 76) = 16.32, p < .01$; for question, $F(3, 228) = 10.96, p < .01$; and for category type, $F(5, 380) = 50.81, p < .01$. The following interactions were also significant: group × question, $F(9, 228) = 30.76, p < .01$; group × category type, $F(15, 380) = 6.22, p < .01$; question × category type, $F(15, 1,140) = 53.16, p < .01$; and group × question × category type, $F(45, 1,140) = 7.06, p < .01$.

As hypothesized, a comparison of means (see Table 3) revealed both cultural and socioeconomic differences in the types of descriptors used by mothers in response to the open-ended questions, with cultural differences emerging most clearly in relation to adult socialization goals, and socioeconomic differences with reference to child behavior. In particular, consistent with their more individualistic cultural orientation, both groups of Anglo mothers were more likely than both Puerto Rican groups to use Self-Maximization when describing desirable adult behavior. (Category usage throughout these studies includes responses indicating either that a behavior was liked because it demonstrated the desirable quality in question [e.g., independence], or disliked because it failed to demonstrate that quality [e.g., clinginess]). In contrast, in keeping with their more sociocentric cultural orientation, both Puerto Rican groups were more likely than both Anglo groups to use Proper Demeanor when describing undesirable adult behavior. Other cultural differences arose, but varied across socioeconomic status (e.g., middle-class but not working-class Anglo mothers were more likely than both Puerto Rican groups to use Self-Maximization when describing desirable child behavior).

Culture and Socioeconomic Status

To further investigate the relative influence of culture and socioeconomic status on group differences in the use of the five content categories for each of the four open-ended questions, hierarchical regression analyses were performed using cultural membership (Anglo vs. Puerto Rican) and Hollingshead score simultaneously as variables.[3]

[3]Because of Puerto Rico's long-standing formal participation in the U.S. economy first as a territory and then as a legal commonwealth of the United States, as well as the extent to which its educational system has been modeled after that of the United States, socioeconomic status is considered roughly comparable across the two groups using Hollingshead's (1975) scaling instrument.

TABLE 3. Mean Percentages of Category Usage, Open-Ended Conceptualizations, Study 1

Category	Anglo		Puerto Rican	
	Middle	Working	Middle	Working
	Positive adult characteristics			
Self-Maximization[a]	64.5%	50.9%	23.3%	14.1%
Self-Control	4.7%	5.9%	3.6%	0.6%
Lovingness	14.7%	9.8%	17.3%	9.5%
Decency	6.6%	13.7%	19.9%	15.4%
Proper Demeanor	8.7%	19.2%	35.5%	60.3%
Miscellaneous	0.9%	0.5%	0.2%	0.1%
	Negative adult characteristics			
Self-Maximization	26.2%	18.6%	10.5%	6.8%
Miscellaneous	0.7%	0.7%	0.4%	0.1%
Self-Control	38.0%	24.6%	18.4%	0.9%
Lovingness	12.0%	11.0%	10.8%	3.5%
Decency	5.9%	25.1%	11.4%	15.1%
Proper Demeanor[a]	17.2%	20.0%	48.4%	73.6%
Miscellaneous	10.7%	0.7%	0.4%	0.1%
	Positive child characteristics			
Self-Maximization	53.9%	36.9%	24.6%	6.1%
Self-Control	5.0%	4.0%	2.3%	0.0%
Lovingness	24.0%	11.9%	26.6%	18.6%
Decency	2.7%	4.3%	10.0%	16.4%
Proper Demeanor[b]	13.2%	41.4%	36.2%	59.0%
Miscellaneous	1.3%	1.5%	0.5%	0.0%
	Negative child characteristics			
Self-Maximization	33.7%	11.4%	9.5%	1.8%
Self-Control	32.9%	37.0%	28.2%	15.1%
Lovingness	6.1%	3.5%	10.2%	2.5%
Decency	5.2%	5.1%	6.1%	3.9%
Proper Demeanor[b]	21.8%	42.7%	45.8%	76.7%
Miscellaneous	0.3%	0.3%	0.0%	0.0%

Note. Categories in Table 3 do not add up to 100% because of rounding. Analyses were performed on transformed means, but tables present untransformed means.
[a]For cultural differences (both Anglo groups compared to both Puerto Rican groups), $p < .01$.
[b]For class differences (both middle-class groups compared to both working-class groups), $p < .01$.

As can be seen in Table 4, the squared semipartial correlations of this analysis indicate that both culture and socioeconomic status contributed significantly to the variance in category usage. However, culture appeared to be the more consistent predictor with regard to adult socialization goals, whereas socioeconomic status as indexed by Hollingshead score emerged more clearly as a major predictor of descriptions of child behavior. In particular, culture was the major significant predictor for group differences in the use of the following categories: Self-Maximization for desirable and undesirable adult characteristics and desirable child characteristics; Self-Control for undesirable adult and desirable child characteristics; Decency for desirable child characteristics; and Proper Demeanor for desirable and undesirable adult characteristics.

Socioeconomic status contributed to most of the variance in category usage in four instances: Lovingness, desirable and undesirable child characteristics; Decency, undesirable adult characteristics; and Proper Demeanor, desirable child characteristics. In addition, culture and socioeconomic status contributed roughly equal proportions of variance in two categories describing undesirable child characteristics: Self-Maximization and Proper Demeanor.

In all, culture contributed to most of the variance in 57% of the 14 analyses for which significant predictors emerged (five adult socialization categories, and three child behavior categories). Socioeconomic status as indexed by Hollingshead score was the major predictor in 19% of the analyses for which significant predictors emerged (one adult socialization and three child behavior categories). As mentioned above, culture and socioeconomic status also emerged as strong copredictors in two categories describing undesirable child behavior.

These results suggest that Kohn's (1977) findings regarding socioeconomic status and the relative valuing of autonomy and conformity may be most relevant to parents' views on child behavior. This finding is in accord with the method Kohn used to elicit his results—a method that involved asking parents to identify the qualities most important for a child of a specific age to possess. Cultural values, on the other hand, may be more evident when parents are considering long-term socialization goals.

Although socioeconomic influences emerged more strongly in relation to child behavior, culture was overall the most consistent predictor of group differences. This finding receives additional support from Kohn's (1977) study of socioeconomic differences in Italy and

TABLE 4. Hierarchical Regression Analyses, Culture and Socioeconomic Status (Hollingshead Score), Open-Ended Conceptualizations, Study 1

Category	Predictor	Semipartial R^2
	Positive adult characteristics	
Self-Maximization	Culture	.37**
	SES	.03*
Self-Control	No variable met conventional significance levels	
Lovingness	No variable met conventional significance levels	
Decency	No variable met conventional significance levels	
Proper Demeanor	Culture	.29**
	SES	.10**
	Negative adult characteristics	
Self-Maximization	Culture	.11**
Self-Control	Culture	.15**
	SES	.10**
Lovingness	No variable met conventional significance levels	
Decency	SES	.08*
Proper Demeanor	Culture	.33**
	SES	.05*
	Positive child characteristics	
Self-Maximization	Culture	.24**
	SES	.08**
Self-Control	Culture	.06*
Lovingness	SES	.06*
Decency	Culture	.09**
Proper Demeanor	SES	.20**
	Culture	.06*
	Negative child characteristics	
Self-Maximization	Culture	.10**
	SES	.09**
Self-Control	No variable met conventional significance levels	
Lovingness	SES	.05*
Decency	No variable met conventional significance levels	
Proper Demeanor	SES	.16**
	Culture	.15**

Note. Regression analyses were performed using transformed means. Regression analyses were not performed on the Miscellaneous category because of the small percentage of responses falling into this category. Significance levels for entry into the model were set at .15, but only variables reaching less than .05 are included in the table.
*$p < .05$.
**$p < .01$.

the United States, in which it was found that although socioeconomic groups differed in both cultures in the predicted direction, differences between the two countries were nonetheless greater than socioeconomic differences within each country.

Sociodemographic Characteristics

Covariate Analyses

Analyses of covariance were undertaken in order to determine whether the effects of culture on mothers' open-ended conceptualizations would change when other sociodemographic characteristics were taken into consideration. In particular, analyses of covariance were performed on seven maternal characteristics (age, education, marital status, total number of children, employment status, number of hours worked outside the home, and economic self-sufficiency as determined by welfare status), and two child characteristics (target child's sex and age). The analyses revealed that the effects of culture remained significant when the demographic characteristics were covaried, suggesting that the effects of culture cannot be reduced to a variety of component sociodemographic characteristics. However, although differences in culture cannot be reduced to differences in sociodemographic characteristics, it was also evident from the analyses that many of these characteristics produced their own independent effects.

Stepwise Regression Analyses

To clarify the relative contributions of culture and sociodemographic characteristics to group differences in the use of the five content categories for each of the four open-ended questions, we used stepwise regression analyses. With these analyses we generated best-fit models for culture and 14 sociodemographic characteristics falling into three categories: (1) socioeconomic characteristics, including Hollingshead occupational prestige score, maternal and paternal education, and welfare status; (2) other sociodemographic characteristics, including household size and composition, total number of children, marital status, maternal age, and three indices of maternal employment [working outside home or not, employed full-time or not, number of hours worked per week]; and (3) target child's age and sex. In the stepwise regressions, all 15 variables were entered into one equation as predictors of mothers' use of each content category for each of the four open-ended questions (desirable and undesirable adult socialization goals, desirable and undesirable child behavior).

As can be seen in Table 5, the results indicate that culture was again the most consistent major contributor to variance in category usage; however, this tendency was again more pronounced with regard to adult socialization goals than it was in relation to child behavior. In particular, culture was the major significant predictor for group differences in the use of the following categories: Self-Maximization for desirable and undesirable adult characteristics and desirable child characteristics; Self-Control for undesirable adult and desirable child characteristics; Decency for desirable child characteristics; and Proper Demeanor for desirable and undesirable adult characteristics.

Socioeconomic characteristics contributed to most of the variance in category usage in five instances: Lovingness, undesirable adult and desirable child characteristics; Decency, undesirable adult characteristics; and Proper Demeanor, desirable and undesirable child characteristics. Other sociodemographic characteristics contributed to most of the variance in four instances: Self-Control, desirable adult and undesirable child characteristics; and Decency, desirable child (copredictor) and undesirable child characteristics.

In all, culture contributed to most of the variance in 55% of the 18 analyses for which significant predictors emerged (six of nine adult socialization categories, and four of nine child behavior categories, including one copredictor). Socioeconomic variables were the major predictors in 28% of the analyses (two adult socialization and three child behavior categories). Other sociodemographic characteristics (household size, household composition, target child's age, and marital status) emerged as major predictors in 22% of the analyses (one adult and three child behavior categories, including one copredictor).

Summary of Open-Ended Conceptualizations

Together, these results suggest that culture, socioeconomic status, and sociodemographic characteristics contributed independently to group differences in mothers' open-ended conceptualizations regarding desirable and undesirable attachment behavior. The regression results

TABLE 5. Stepwise Regression Analyses, Sociodemographic Characteristics, Open-Ended Conceptualizations, Study 1

Category	Predictor	Semipartial R^2
	Positive adult characteristics	
Self-Maximization	Culture	.45**
	Household size	.04*
Self-Control	Household size	.07*
Lovingness	No variable met conventional significance levels	
Decency	Culture	.14**
	No. hours worked/week	.06*
Proper Demeanor	Culture	.33**
	Maternal employment status	.16**
	Negative adult characteristics	
Self-Maximization	Culture	.13**
Self-Control	Culture	.20**
Lovingness	Father's education	.09*
Decency	Father's education	.18**
	Marital status	.09*
Proper Demeanor	Culture	.37**
	Household size	.11**
	Positive child characteristics	
Self-Maximization	Culture	.29**
	Hollingshead score	.14**
Self-Control	Culture	.10*
Lovingness	Welfare status	.07*
	Child's age	.07*
Decency	Culture	.08*
	Household composition	.08*
Proper Demeanor	Hollingshead score	.29**
	Child's age	.08*
	Negative child characteristics	
Self-Maximization	Culture	.17**
	Mother's education	.08*
Self-Control	Child's age	.14**
Lovingness	No variable met conventional significance levels	
Decency	Marital status	.10*
Proper Demeanor	Mother's education	.21**
	Culture	.13**

Note. Regression analyses were performed using transformed means. Regression analyses were not performed on the Miscellaneous category because of the small percentage of responses falling into this category. Significance levels for entry into the model were set at .15, but only variables reaching less than .05 are included in the table.
*$p < .05$.
**$p < .01$.

suggest that culture was overall the major predictor of group variance in mothers' meaning systems, particularly when long-term socialization goals were considered. In contrast, socioeconomic and other sociodemographic variables emerged most strongly as major predictors in category usage in the descriptions of child behaivor.

Culturally Sensitive Strange Situation Behaviors

Coding Categories

In order to create culturally sensitive vignettes of desirable and undesirable Strange Situation behavior, mothers' descriptions in response to questions 5a–5c and 6a–6c of first a desirable and then an undesirable toddler in a simulated Strange Situation were coded into 34 categories representing behavior in each of the three major episodes of the Strange Situation: preseparation, separation, and reunion. These 34 categories were based on an exhaustive analysis of mothers' descriptions of desirable and undesirable Strange Situation behavior, and represented all examples generated by the mothers.

Because culturally sensitive vignettes had already been created for use with a working-class migrant Puerto Rican population (Harwood, 1992), of interest in Study 1 was whether these vignettes would also capture culturally relevant concerns of middle- and working-class island Puerto Rican mothers. In order to examine this, the behavioral coding categories were combined into seven dimensions: (1) Balance of Play and Relatedness (playing at a distance and involving the mother during the preseparation episode; playing happily during at least part of the separation episode; and greeting the mother happily and approaching her for contact during the reunion episode); (2) Respectfulness (sitting near the mother, sitting before approaching toys, waiting for a parental signal before playing, and playing quietly during preseparation; and waiting quietly for the mother to return during separation); (3) Clinginess (clinging to the mother during preseparation, crying the whole time without playing during separation, and being unhappy during the reunion); (4) Avoidance (ignoring the mother during all three episodes); (5) Aggression (aggressive behavior—i.e., hitting and throwing things at people—during preseparation and separation); (6) Expresses Anger (temper tantrum during separation and expression of anger on reunion); and (7) Activity Level (highly active during each of the three episodes).

Analysis of Strange Situation Category Usage

Fisher exact tests were performed on the frequencies of mothers' responses that could be coded into each of these seven category clusters. As can be seen in Table 6, compared to the Puerto Rican mothers, the Anglo mothers used Balance of Play and Relatedness more often to describe desirable Strange Situation behavior, and Clinginess more often to describe undesirable Strange Situation behavior. In contrast, the Puerto Rican mothers used Respectfulness more often to describe desirable behavior, and Activity Level and Avoidance more often to describe undesirable behavior. No cultural differences occurred in the use of the categories of Aggressiveness and Expresses Anger.

It thus appeared that the same behavioral dimensions that had proven most salient for migrant mothers also emerged as important to the island mothers. It was therefore decided that the culturally sensitive vignettes created in Harwood (1992) for use with migrant Puerto Rican mothers were appropriate for use with island mothers as well. In addition, the results of this analysis provide further confirmation of cultural differences in mothers' perceptions of desirable and undesirable Strange Situation behavior: Anglo mothers preferred that toddlers balance autonomy and relatedness, and they disliked clinginess; Puerto Rican mothers preferred that toddlers display respectfulness, and they disliked highly active or avoidant behaviors.

STUDY 2: EVALUATION OF ATTACHMENT BEHAVIOR

The purpose of Study 2 was to examine the impact of cultural values on mothers' evaluations of attachment behavior, using vignettes of Strange Situation behavior indigenous to both Anglo and Puerto Rican

TABLE 6. Frequencies of Usage of Strange Situation Behavioral Categories

Behavioral category	Anglo	Puerto Rican	p^a
Balance of Play and Relatedness	4.28	3.0	.0002
Respectfulness	0.65	1.5	.008
Activity Level	0.38	1.25	.00004
Clinginess	2.38	1.45	.013
Avoidance	1.23	2.0	.00007
Aggression	0.68	0.60	n.s.
Expresses Anger	0.83	0.65	n.s.

[a]Significance was computed using Fisher exact test.

mothers. Because the dimensions of Strange Situation behavior that had been identified by Harwood (1992) as important to working-class migrant Puerto Rican mothers also emerged as salient to middle- and working-class island mothers, the island groups were administered the same protocol that was administered in Harwood (1992). The six vignettes used in Study 2 are provided in the Appendix.

Study Participants

As in Study 1, comparison was undertaken of the conceptualizations of middle- and working-class mainland Anglo mothers, and middle- and working-class island Puerto Rican mothers (n = 20 for each group). Mothers were drawn from the same geographical regions as in Study 1, and had at least one child aged 12–24 months—the age during which quality of attachment is normally assessed using the Strange Situation (Ainsworth et al., 1978). There were no differences in the age of the Strange Situation-age children across the four groups (mean = 17.7 months), and gender distribution was equal.

Demographically, the groups used in Study 2 were similar to those used in Study 1 (see Table 7). Among the two middle-class groups, Puerto Rican mothers were younger than Anglo mothers, and more likely to be employed outside the home (95% of the Puerto Rican

TABLE 7. Demographic Characteristics, Study 2

	Middle-class		Working-class	
Characteristic	Anglo	Puerto Rican	Anglo	Puerto Rican
Target child's age (months)	17.2	16.3	17.8	19.6
Mother's age	32.3	28.8*	27.2	26.0
Mother's education (years)	16.5	16.0	11.7	9.8**
% mothers employed[a]	65.0	95.0*	15.0	0.0
% working full-time	35.0	37.0	0.0	0.0
No. of hours worked per week	21.9	23.7	1.6	0.0
% married	95.0	90.0	45.0	60.0
Total no. of children	1.5	1.6	2.1	2.0
Household size (no. of people)	3.5	3.5	4.1	4.5
Father's education	17.1	15.9	12.0	9.8**
Hollingshead score	57.0	54.1	23.6	13.7**
% on AFDC (welfare)	—	—	100.0	100.0

Note. n = 20 in each group.
[a]Significance was computed using Fisher exact test.
*p < .05.
**p < .01.

mothers, compared to 65% of the Anglo mothers, had jobs). Among the two working-class groups, Anglo mothers were better educated than Puerto Rican mothers, as were their husbands if present. In addition, Anglo working-class mothers were more likely to be living in a household in which there was an employed adult present (only one of the Puerto Rican working-class mothers was living in a wage-earning household, compared to 65% of the Anglo mothers). These differences in education and employment status produced higher Hollingshead scores for the Anglo mothers than for the Puerto Rican mothers (respective means were 23.6 and 13.7).

Significant demographic differences between the two middle-class groups and between the two working-class groups may represent either sampling error or differences in the larger societal contexts. Within-class differences that are consistent across the two studies would suggest differences in the larger societal contexts, whereas within-class differences that are unique to either Study 1 or Study 2 would suggest the presence of sampling error. Among the two middle-class groups across both Studies 1 and 2, Puerto Rican mothers were younger than Anglo mothers; there was no other demographic variable on which the two middle-class samples differed across both studies, and all middle-class mothers were recruited through university communities. These results suggest that either (1) the University of Puerto Rico attracts younger female populations than does Yale University; or (2) middle-class professional Puerto Rican women may be choosing to start their families at a younger age than their Anglo counterparts. The national trends within the mainland United States for delayed childbearing among highly educated, professional women suggest that the latter argument may have some merit.

There were no differences between the two working-class groups that occurred across both studies. However, the working-class Puerto Rican sample employed in Study 2 was poorer and less educated than the working-class Puerto Rican sample used in Study 1. In order to assess the impact of this sample difference, a measure of adult socialization goals was administered to all Study 2 participants to test for comparability of cultural value systems among mothers across the two studies.

Procedures Used

Study 2 consisted of both closed and open-ended assessments of six hypothetical toddlers (see the Appendix). These assessments were

based on the culturally sensitive descriptions of desirable and undesirable Strange Situation behavior, constructed into vignettes on the
basis of mothers' responses in Harwood (1992).

Vignettes

Again, the Strange Situation was chosen for the investigation of mothers' perceptions of attachment behavior because it is both standardized and widely used. At least two methodological options exist: It is
possible to present mothers either with verbal descriptions of Strange
Situation behavior in the form of vignettes, or with brief clips from
videos of actual Strange Situation assessments. The first option was
chosen because, besides permitting "tailor-made" descriptions of culturally sensitive desirable and undesirable Strange Situation behavior, it also allowed greater standardization of toddler behavior across
ethnic groups, permitted greater control of focal attention, and reduced
information-processing demands on subjects.

It must be noted that Ainsworth's classifications are flexible
enough to allow for behavioral variations within each of the three
broad classifications, as well as within the paradigm's eight subclassifications. It is thus impossible to create a single toddler whose character is prototypically representative of each attachment classification
or subclassification. Instead, one must be aware that a range of behaviors falls within each of the Group A, B, and C classifications. Each
of the six hypothetical toddlers portrayed in this study represents just
one instance of six of the eight attachment subclassifications: A1
(highly avoidant), B1 and B2 (the "distal" Bs), B3 and B4 (the "proximal" Bs), and C1 (extremely clingy and angry); however, they represent characterizations possessing a high degree of salience for the different groups of mothers.

Open-Ended and Closed Assessments

After an assessment of the Study 2 subjects' comparability to Study 1
subjects (see below), subjects listened to and responded to six vignettes,
each describing the behavior of one hypothetical 18-month-old toddler left briefly with an unfamiliar adult in an unfamiliar setting (the
waiting room of a doctor's office). Each vignette described the toddler's
behavior during three separate episodes: preseparation, separation, and
reunion. The vignettes thus sought to simulate the primary characteristics of the Strange Situation. The sex of the children portrayed in

the vignettes was matched to the sex of each subject's attachment-age child; the vignettes were presented to subjects in randomized orders.

Mothers looked at a drawing of the setting of a Strange Situation (see Figure 1, above; Harwood, 1992), while the interviewers read to them the vignettes describing the behavior of each of the hypothetical toddlers. Following each story, mothers' open-ended conceptualizations of each of the toddlers were elicited. After each mother's open-ended reactions were obtained, the mother completed a rating task assessing her perceptions of the relative desirability, typicality, and similarity to her own attachment-age child of each of the six hypothetical toddlers. To reduce response bias, mothers rated desirability in conjunction with the open-ended questions, but rated typicality and similarity after hearing all the vignettes.

In order to minimize literacy and task familiarity effects, mothers were shown a visual representation of a 9-point scale during the rating tasks, and its significance was explained to them. In order to refresh their memories concerning the behavior of each of the hypothetical toddlers, mothers were invited to read each of the vignettes before completing the rating tasks, and were also reminded orally of their descriptions of each of the six toddlers. The questionnaire was administered orally and took about an hour to complete.

A Spanish version of the questionnaire was prepared for use with the Puerto Rican mothers. This translation was undertaken by native speakers of Puerto Rican Spanish, employing back-translation techniques. Interviews with the mothers were administered individually by ethnically matched, trained interviewers.

Comparability Assessment. In order to insure that mothers' socialization values were similar to those of subjects in Study 1, all mothers were asked at the beginning of the interview the first two questions that had been asked of mothers in Study 1:

1. "Most mothers, when they have a child, have some idea about what sorts of qualities they would like their children to possess—what kind of person they would like their children to grow up to be. When you think about your children, what sorts of qualities would you like them to possess as they grow older?"

2. "Again, most mothers have some idea about what sorts of qualities they would really *not* like their children to possess. When you think about your children, what sorts of qualities would you *not* want them to possess as they grow older?"

Open-Ended Conceptualizations of Toddlers. After listening to each vignette, subjects answered two questions designed to assess their open-ended conceptualizations of each toddler:

3. "Let's assume that [name]'s behavior in this story is typical of his/her behavior in general. How would you describe his/her personality?"
4. "Why would or wouldn't you want your own child to act this way in the same situation?"

Subjects' open-ended conceptualizations were analyzed according to the same procedure used in Study 1 into the same categories, with the exception that the Decency category was not used because it was not pertinent to toddler behavior. Again, the categories used were as follows: Self-Maximization, or a toddler's ability to demonstrate self-confidence, independence, and the development of his or her talents as an individual; Self-Control, or a toddler's ability to curb negative impulses toward greed, egocentrism, and aggression; Lovingness, or a toddler's ability to be loving and affectionate; Proper Demeanor, or a toddler's ability to be well mannered, well behaved, cooperative, and accepted by the larger community, and the parents' corresponding ability to perform their parental duties appropriately; and Miscellaneous, a fifth category containing all content responses that could not be coded in the first four categories. Fewer than 5% of all content responses were coded into the Miscellaneous category across all five groups. Reliability in coding mothers' open-ended conceptualizations of the six hypothetical toddlers was calculated between the first author (Harwood) and an independent judge on 50% of the interviews. Overall agreement reached a level of .93 (Cohen's kappa).

Perceived Desirability, Typicality, and Similarity Ratings. Mothers rated the following statements on a 9-point scale, ranging from "extremely no" (1) to "extremely yes" (9): "How much would you like your own child to act this way in the same situation?" (desirability); "Most 18-month-old toddlers would act like this in a similar situation" (typicality); and "My own child acts like this in a similar situation" (similarity).

Analyses

As in Study 1, preliminary analyses revealed significant group differences in the total number of descriptors generated by subjects

$(p < .01)$. To control for these differences, subsequent analyses focused on the percentages rather than on the frequencies of descriptors generated by mothers. Also as in Study 1, subsequent analyses employed arc–sine transformations appropriate for use with proportional data.

Comparability Assessment

Mothers' responses to the first two questions were analyzed according to the same procedure used in Study 1, using the same six categories: Self-Maximization, Self-Control, Lovingness, Proper Demeanor, Decency, and Miscellaneous. A $4 \times 2 \times 6$ (group × question × category type) ANOVA was performed on the relative percentages of subjects' descriptors that could be coded into each of the categories. As in Study 1, this ANOVA yielded a significant main effect for category type, $F(5, 380) = 48.59$, $p < .01$, as well as significant interactions of group × question, $F(3, 380) = 29.14$, $p < .01$; group × category type, $F(15, 380) = 4.1$, $p < .01$; question × category type, $F(5, 380) = 24.78$, $p < .01$; and group × question × category type, $F(15, 380) = 5.13$, $p < .01$.

A post hoc comparison of means revealed trends similar to those found for questions 1 and 2 in Study 1, suggesting that the two samples of mothers were comparable in their value systems regarding desirable and undesirable adult socialization goals. In particular, as in Study 1, both middle- and working-class Anglo mothers, compared to both middle- and working-class Puerto Rican mothers, were more likely to generate desirable adult descriptors that could be coded into the category of Self-Maximization, and less likely to generate desirable and undesirable adult descriptors that could be coded into the category of Proper Demeanor. Social class differences also emerged but were not consistent across culture (see Table 8). Moreover, as in Study 1, hierarchical regressions (see Table 9) analyzing the relative contribution to these results of culture and 14 sociodemographic variables indicated that culture contributed to most of the variance in the use of Self-Maximization and Proper Demeanor when mothers were describing both desirable and undesirable adult behavior.

Open-Ended Conceptualizations of Toddlers

To compare subjects' open-ended conceptualizations of each hypothetical toddler, a $4 \times 6 \times 5$ (group × toddler × category type) ANOVA

TABLE 8. Comparability Assessment, Open-Ended Conceptualizations, Study 2

	Anglo		Puerto Rican	
Category	Middle	Working	Middle	Working
	Positive adult characteristics			
Self-Maximization[a]	48.5%	47.1%	18.4%	25.4%
Self-Control	3.5%	1.5%	2.1%	0.7%
Lovingness	27.7%	16.4%	12.4%	4.1%
Decency	10.3%	18.4%	28.1%	15.2%
Proper Demeanor[a]	8.7%	15.4%	38.9%	44.0%
Miscellaneous	1.3%	1.3%	0.0%	0.7%
	Negative adult characteristics			
Self-Maximization	17.6%	20.1%	5.7%	2.1%
Self-Control	52.3%	21.5%	15.4%	10.5%
Lovingness	11.2%	2.3%	1.1%	3.9%
Decency	12.7%	34.8%	26.9%	31.3%
Proper Demeanor[a]	5.7%	21.3%	49.2%	52.2%
Miscellaneous	0.4%	0.0%	1.7%	0.0%

Note. Categories in Table 8 do not add up to 100% because of rounding. Analyses were performed on transformed means, but tables present untransformed means.
[a]For cultural differences (both Anglo groups compared to both Puerto Rican groups), $p < .01$.

was performed on the relative percentages of subjects' descriptors that could be coded into each of the categories. This ANOVA yielded significant main effects for toddler, $F (5, 380) = 39.16, p < .01$, and category type, $F (4, 304) = 181.89, p < .01$. The following interactions were also significant: group × toddler, $F (15, 380) = 3.76, p < .01$; group × category type, $F (12, 304) = 37.28, p < .01$; toddler × category type, $F (20, 1,520) = 28.35, p < .01$; and group × toddler × category type, $F (60, 1520) = 4.92, p < .01$.

A comparison of means revealed significant group differences in the types of descriptors used by mothers. As hypothesized, compared to both Puerto Rican groups, both Anglo groups were more likely to describe four of the six toddlers in terms of Self-Maximization, and less likely to evaluate four of the six toddlers in terms of Proper Demeanor (see Table 10). Other significant cultural differences occurred, but varied with socioeconomic status.

Social class differences also emerged, but were consistent across both cultural groups in just one instance: working-class mothers were more likely than middle-class mothers to use the Proper Demeanor category when describing the A1 toddler.

TABLE 9. Hierarchical Regression Analyses, Culture and Socioeconomic Status, Open-Ended Conceptualizations, Study 2

Category	Predictor	Semipartial R^2
	Positive adult characteristics	
Self-Maximization	Culture	.22**
Self-Control	No variable met conventional significance levels	
Lovingness	Culture	.05*
Decency	No variable met conventional significance levels	
Proper Demeanor	Culture	.22**
	Negative adult characteristics	
Self-Maximization	Culture	.13**
Self-Control	Culture	.13**
	SES	.04*
Lovingness	No variable met conventional significance levels	
Decency	Hollingshead score	.05*
Proper Demeanor	Culture	.20**

Note. Regression analyses were performed using transformed means. Regression analyses were not performed on the Miscellaneous category because of the small percentage of responses falling into this category. Significance levels for entry into the model were set at .15, but only variables reaching less than .05 are included in the table.
*$p < .05$.
**$p < .01$.

Culture and Socioeconomic Status

To further investigate the relative influence of culture and socioeconomic status on group differences in the use of the four content categories when mothers described each of the six hypothetical toddlers, we performed a hierarchical regression analysis using cultural membership (Anglo vs. Puerto Rican) and Hollingshead score entered simultaneously as variables.

As can be seen in Table 11, the squared semipartial correlations of this analysis indicate that culture was the major contributor to most of the variance in the use of Self-Maximization for all but the C1 toddler, and Proper Demeanor for all six toddlers. In addition, culture was the major predictor for mothers' use of the following categories: Self-Control when describing the B2, B3, and C1 toddlers; and Lovingness when describing the B2 and B3 toddlers.

Socioeconomic status as indexed by Hollingshead score contributed to most of the variance in the use of the Lovingness category for the B1 and C1 toddlers, and was a strong copredictor for the use of the Lovingness category for the A1 toddler.

TABLE 10. Mean Percentages of Category Usage for Open-Ended Conceptualizations of Toddlers

Category	Anglo		Puerto Rican	
	Middle	Working	Middle	Working
	A1 toddler			
Self-Maximization[a]	59.2%	48.2%	19.6%	4.9%
Self-Control	3.0%	8.2%	4.3%	2.8%
Lovingness	27.9%	13.0%	11.7%	2.4%
Proper Demeanor[a]	10.0%	29.1%	64.4%	88.1%
Miscellaneous	0.0%	1.5%	0.0%	1.7%
	B1 toddler			
Self-Maximization[a]	73.0%	70.6%	37.2%	19.7%
Self-Control	1.9%	0.6%	2.5%	11.5%
Lovingness	17.9%	9.0%	11.3%	3.2%
Proper Demeanor[a]	6.9%	19.0%	49.0%	65.5%
Miscellaneous	0.4%	0.7%	0.0%	0.0%
	B2 toddler			
Self-Maximization[b]	64.1%	63.9%	46.5%	37.6%
Self-Control	2.5%	3.0%	1.2%	0.0%
Lovingness	27.8%	15.3%	9.3%	5.6%
Proper Demeanor[a]	5.2%	16.9%	42.4%	56.8%
Miscellaneous	0.4%	0.9%	0.6%	0.0%
	B3 toddler			
Self-Maximization[b]	56.1%	51.5%	30.8%	3.9%
Self-Control	1.0%	2.4%	0.0%	0.0%
Lovingness	27.4%	22.1%	16.3%	11.1%
Proper Demeanor[a]	15.5%	24.0%	52.2%	84.4%
Miscellaneous	0.0%	0.0%	0.7%	0.6%
	B4 toddler			
Self-Maximization	80.7%	67.8%	62.3%	55.9%
Self-Control	1.6%	10.3%	8.0%	19.5%
Lovingness	11.2%	19.1%	16.4%	11.9%
Proper Demeanor	4.1%	2.9%	12.8%	10.2%
Miscellaneous	2.4%	0.0%	0.6%	2.5%
	C1 toddler			
Self-Maximization	42.0%	29.7%	26.4%	27.9%
Self-Control	37.5%	38.5%	25.5%	17.4%
Lovingness	12.5%	9.6%	13.0%	4.9%
Proper Demeanor	7.4%	20.8%	34.6%	49.8%
Miscellaneous	0.6%	1.5%	0.5%	0.0%

Note. Categories in Table 10 do not add up to 100% because of rounding. Analyses were performed on transformed means, but tables present untransformed means.
[a]For cultural differences (both Anglo groups compared to both Puerto Rican groups), $p < .01$.
[b]For cultural differences, $p < .05$.

TABLE 11. Hierarchical Regression Analyses, Culture and Socioeconomic Status, Open-Ended Conceptualizations of Toddlers

Category	Predictor	Semipartial R^2
	A1 toddler	
Self-Maximization	Culture	.28**
Self-Control	No variables met conventional significance levels	
Lovingness	Culture	.09
	SES	.08**
Proper Demeanor	Culture	.35**
	SES	.04
	B1 toddler	
Self-Maximization	Culture	.29**
Self-Control	No variables met conventional significance levels	
Lovingness	SES	.07
Proper Demeanor	Culture	.24**
	B2 toddler	
Self-Maximization	Culture	.08**
Self-Control	Culture	.10 *
Lovingness	Culture	.09**
Proper Demeanor	Culture	.22**
	B3 toddler	
Self-Maximization	Culture	.12**
	SES	.07**
Self-Control	Culture	.07**
Lovingness	Culture	.07*
Proper Demeanor	Culture	.27**
	SES	.07**
	B4 toddler	
Self-Maximization	Culture	.06**
	SES	.04
Self-Control	No variables met conventional significance levels	
Lovingness	No variables met conventional significance levels	
Proper Demeanor	Culture	.08**
	C1 toddler	
Self-Maximization	No variables met conventional significance levels	
Self-Control	Culture	.11**
Lovingness	SES	.08*
Proper Demeanor	Culture	.20**
	SES	.04**

Note. Regression analyses were performed using transformed means. Regression analyses were not performed on the Miscellaneous category because of the small percentage of responses falling into this category. Significance levels for entry into the model were set at .15, but only variables reaching less than .05 are included in the table.
*$p < .05$.
**$p < .01$.

Sociodemographic Characteristics

Covariate Analyses

As in Study 1, analyses of covariance were undertaken in order to determine whether the effects of culture on mothers' category usage when describing the six toddlers would change when other sociodemographic characteristics were taken into consideration. The analyses revealed that the effects of culture remained significant when seven maternal and two child demographic characteristics were covaried, suggesting that the effects of culture cannot be reduced to a variety of component sociodemographic characteristics. However, although differences in culture cannot be reduced to differences in sociodemographic characteristics, it was again evident from the analyses that many of these characteristics were producing their own independent effects.

Stepwise Regression Analyses

In order to clarify the relative contribution of culture and sociodemographic variables to group differences in category usage when mothers were describing the six hypothetical toddlers, we performed stepwise regression analyses on culture and 14 sociodemographic variables, according to the same procedure described in Study 1. As can be seen in Table 12, the results of the regression analyses indicate that culture was the major contributor to most of the variance in the use of Self-Maximization for all but the C1 toddler, and in the use of the Proper Demeanor category for all six toddlers. In addition, culture was the major predictor for mothers' use of the following categories:

TABLE 12. Stepwise Regression Analyses, Sociodemographic Characteristics, Open-Ended Conceptualizations of Toddlers

Category	Predictor	Partial R^2
	A1 toddler	
Self-Maximization	Culture	.39**
Self-Control	Culture	.39**
Lovingness	Culture	.16**
	Maternal employment status	.07*
Proper Demeanor	Culture	.52**
	No hours worked/week	.09**

(continued)

TABLE 12 (*continued*)

Category	Predictor	Partial R^2
	B1 toddler	
Self-Maximization	Culture	.44**
Self-Control	Household composition	.11**
Lovingness	No. hours worked/week	.09*
Proper Demeanor	Culture	.39**
	No. hours worked/week	.04*
	B2 toddler	
Self-Maximization	Culture	.11**
Self-Control	Culture	.10 *
Lovingness	Culture	.13**
Proper Demeanor	Culture	.32**
	B3 toddler	
Self-Maximization	Culture	.42**
	Hollingshead score	.07**
Self-Control	Hollingshead score	.11**
Lovingness	Welfare status	.08*
Proper Demeanor	Culture	.49**
	No. hours worked/week	.07**
	B4 toddler	
Self-Maximization	Culture	.15**
Self-Control	Welfare status	.13**
	Household composition	.06*
Lovingness	Household size	.11**
	Child's age	.08*
	No. hours worked/week	.05*
Proper Demeanor	Culture	.16**
	Child's age	.06*
	C1 toddler	
Self-Maximization	Mother's age	.11**
Self-Control	Maternal employment status	.12**
	Mother's age	.07*
	Culture	.06*
Lovingness	Mother's age	.08*
	Marital status	.07**
Proper Demeanor	Culture	.25**
	Father's education	.08**
	Child's age	.05*

Note. Regression analyses were performed using transformed means. Regression analyses were not performed on the Miscellaneous category because of the small percentage of responses falling into this category. Significance levels for entry into the model were set at .15, but only variables reaching less than .05 are included in the table.
*p < .05.
**p < .01.

Self-Control when describing the A1 and B2 toddlers; and Lovingness when describing the A1 and B2 toddlers.

Socioeconomic variables (Hollingshead score and welfare status) contributed to most of the variance in three instances: the use of the Self-Control category for the B3 and B4 toddlers, and the use of the Lovingness category for the B4 toddler. Other sociodemographic characteristics (household size, household composition, mother's age, employment status, and number of hours worked per week) were the major predictors in six instances: the use of the Self-Maximization category for the C1 toddler, the use of the Self-Control category for the B1 and C1 toddlers, and the use of the Lovingness category for the B1, B4, and C1 toddlers.

Perceived Desirability, Typicality, and Similarity

Because a moderate number of significant intercorrelations occurred among the variables of perceived desirability, typicality, and similarity, a multivariate analysis of variance (MANOVA) was deemed the appropriate analysis (33% of the intercorrelations reached conventional levels of significance, with r values ranging from .46 to .77). A $4 \times 6 \times 3$ (group $\times$ toddler $\times$ normative dimensions) repeated-measures MANOVA was performed on mothers' ratings of the hypothetical toddlers' desirability, typicality, and similarity (normative dimensions) to their own target-age child. This MANOVA yielded significant main effects for toddler, $F(5, 72) = 59.83$, lambda $< .01$, and norms, $F(2, 75) = 17.04$, lambda $< .01$. These interactions were also significant: group $\times$ toddler, $F(15, 199) = 2.11$, lambda $< .05$; group $\times$ norms, $F(6, 150) = 6.0$, lambda $< .01$; toddler $\times$ norms, $F(10, 67) = 22.48$, lambda $< .01$; and group $\times$ toddler $\times$ norms, $F(30, 197) = 3.98$, lambda $< .01$.

Follow-up 4×6 (group $\times$ toddler) ANOVAs revealed significant group differences along the dimension of perceived desirability. In particular, this analysis yielded significant main effects for group, $F(3, 76) = 6.65$, $p < .01$, and toddler, $F(5, 380) = 156.16$, $p < .01$, as well as a significant group $\times$ toddler interaction, $F(15, 380) = 7.11$, $p < .01$. No significant group differences emerged with respect to the perceived typicality or similarity of each of the six toddlers.

As anticipated, a comparison of means revealed cultural differences in the perceived desirability of two of the six hypothetical toddlers. As can be seen in Table 13, compared to both Puerto Rican groups, both Anglo groups viewed the active A1 and B1 toddlers as more desirable. In addition, the middle-class Anglo mothers viewed

TABLE 13. Mothers' Mean Ratings of Toddlers' Desirability, Typicality, and Similarity

Toddler	Anglo		Puerto Rican	
	Middle	Working	Middle	Working
Desirability				
A1[a]	5.6	5.0	2.1	2.2
B1[a]	8.2	8.3	5.9	4.2
B2	8.1	8.3	7.5	7.5
B3	7.2	7.8	8.6	8.6
B4	2.6	2.9	2.4	3.7
C1	2.1	1.9	1.9	1.8
Typicality				
A1	3.3	4.7	5.0	4.7
B1	5.2	6.2	6.5	6.6
B2	5.6	5.7	6.2	6.4
B3	5.6	5.9	6.0	6.5
B4	5.0	5.7	5.9	5.4
C1	4.2	4.2	5.5	4.2
Similarity				
A1	2.8	3.2	2.9	4.2
B1	5.6	5.3	4.9	5.2
B2	6.9	5.5	6.4	6.8
B3	5.7	5.3	6.3	7.9
B4	3.4	4.5	4.6	4.7
C1	1.9	3.5	2.7	2.9

[a]For cultural differences (both Puerto Rican groups compared to both Anglo groups), $p < .01$.

the more proximal B3 toddler as less desirable than did the Puerto Rican mothers. No other group differences occurred.

GENERAL SUMMARY OF RESULTS

In summary, the results of these two studies suggest that Group B infants were considered most desirable by all groups, whereas the C1 infant was considered least desirable by all groups. However, Self-Maximization and Proper Demeanor are culturally important categories that distinguished the perceptions of Anglo and Puerto Rican mothers on a fairly consistent basis across socioeconomic status. In addition, sociodemographic differences, as well as group differences in the use of the Lovingness and Self-Control categories, also occurred in complex but variable ways.

In terms of mothers' evaluations of attachment behavior, a comparison of group means found cultural differences across socioeconomic status to be more frequent than socioeconomic differences across culture. In particular, cultural differences emerged across class in the use of Self-Maximization and Proper Demeanor for all but the B4 and C1 toddlers, whereas socioeconomic differences occurred across culture in just one instance: the use of Proper Demeanor for the A1 toddler. Other socioeconomic differences occurred but were not consistent across cultural groups.

The stepwise regression analyses on mothers' evaluations of attachment behavior indicated that culture was the most consistent predictor of category usage for all toddlers. In particular, culture contributed to most of the variance for the use of *all* categories for the A1 and B2 toddlers; the use of Proper Demeanor for all toddlers; and the use of Self-Maximization for all but the C1 toddler.

Socioeconomic and other demographic variables were the major predictors of group differences in the use of Self-Control and Lovingness for all but the A1 and B2 toddlers. In all, culture contributed to most of the variance in 15 out of 24 (62.5%) analyses, whereas sociodemographic characteristics contributed to most of the variance in only nine (37.5%) analyses.

Finally, cultural but not socioeconomic differences emerged in mothers' mean ratings of the relative desirability of the hypothetical toddlers. In particular, both groups of Anglo mothers, compared to both groups of Puerto Rican mothers, rated the active A1 and B1 toddlers as more desirable. It could be argued that differences in perceived desirability merely reflect a differential frequency of these patterns in the groups sampled. However, the lack of any group differences in the perceived typicality of the toddlers or their perceived similarity to the mothers' own Strange Situation-age children argues against a one-to-one relationship between judgments of desirability and judgments of similarity or typicality.

Taken together, these findings provide evidence that culture and socioeconomic status contribute independently to findings of group differences in long-term socialization goals, perceptions of child behavior, and the evaluation of attachment behavior. Moreover, when considered together, cultural membership appears to provide a broader basis for group differences than do a variety of sociodemographic characteristics, including multiple socioeconomic indices. The study results thus lend support to the idea that culture constitutes the general meaning systems or "cognitive maps" (see Spradley, 1972) through which the actions of self and others are understood and organized; sociodemographic characteristics may provide junctures for the transformation of those meaning systems into specific, localized variations based, among other things, on economic opportunity and differential access to power and resources. In particular, the consistency with which cultural membership differentiates Anglo and Puerto Rican mothers' usages of the Self-Maximization and Proper Demeanor categories suggests that these two categories may represent central cultural constructs that provide such general meaning systems: Self-Maximization for the Anglo mothers, and Proper Demeanor for the Puerto Rican mothers. In contrast, mothers' usages of the Self-Control and Lovingness categories appear more contextually variable.

It must be emphasized that the present research does not invalidate claims for either the meaningfulness or the predictive significance of individual differences in attachment behavior (Ainsworth et al., 1978). Instead, these findings suggest that we need culturally sensitive models of how that meaningfulness might best be conceptualized in different cultural contexts. Moreover, such culturally sensitive models need to include a consideration of both larger cultural concerns and more localized transformations of those concerns in order to arrive at a fuller understanding of child development in context. We discuss our findings in greater depth in the following chapters.

CHAPTER FOUR

Images of the Child: Autonomy and Relatedness

◆

It has become increasingly common in psychology to describe dominant U.S. culture as individualistic. In particular, Anglo-American culture is generally considered to stress values associated with individualism, such as self-confidence, individual achievement, and independence. Individualism has been treated as a primary analytic dimension of U.S. culture in numerous works, including philosophical and historical treatments of the moral and political status of individual autonomy (Dumont, 1986; Dworkin, 1988; Tuan, 1982); content analyses of person description and explanation (Shweder & Bourne, 1984; J. G. Miller, 1984); observational studies of parent–infant interactions, as well as of teacher–child interactions in a preschool setting (Ochs & Schieffelin, 1984; Tobin, Wu, & Davidson, 1989); linguistic analyses of conversational storytelling and narrative structures in parent–child communications (P. J. Miller, Mintz, Hoogstra, Fung, & Potts, 1992; Polanyi, 1989); cross-cultural and ethnographic studies of values and behaviors (Bellah, Madsen, Sullivan, Swidler, & Tipton, 1985; Harwood, 1992; J. G. Miller & Bersoff, 1992; Lucca, 1988); the examination of culturally based cognitive models of behavior and motivation (D'Andrade, 1992; Harkness, Super, & Keefer, 1992; Strauss, 1992); theoretical expositions on cultural psychology (Markus & Kitayama, 1991; J. G. Miller, 1994; Shweder, 1990); and reflective essays on the history, problems, and potential of psychology as a discipline (Cushman, 1990, 1991; Kessen, 1979; Lasch, 1978; Sampson, 1989; Spence, 1985).

In this chapter, we explore the construct of individualism as it emerged in the responses of both middle- and working-class Anglo mothers to questions regarding their child-rearing goals and values, as well as to the behaviors of hypothetical toddlers in a situation designed to simulate the primary characteristics of the Strange Situation. Although differences according to socioeconomic status did occur among the Anglo mothers, these are discussed in Chapter Six; the present chapter focuses on within-group commonalities rather than within-group variability. Of particular interest in this examination is the extent to which Anglo mothers from a wide range of socioeconomic backgrounds appeared concerned with finding a balance between an overly isolative autonomy and an overly enmeshed relatedness. The successful negotiation of self–other boundaries, leading to the ability to be both self-reliant and open to relationships with others, was viewed as a central task of socialization, and desirable versus undesirable attachment behavior was conceptualized largely in these terms.

MAXIMIZATION OF THE SELF
AS AN AUTONOMOUS UNIT

We chose the term Self-Maximization to refer to one of the major dimensions used by the Anglo mothers in our studies to describe qualities they would like their children to possess as adults, as well as qualities they found desirable in children. This dimension contains three primary interrelated components: (1) independence or self-reliance; (2) self-confidence or a sense of subjective satisfaction; and (3) the development of the individual's full potential in terms of intellect, verbal facility, skills, abilities, and career goals. Somewhat unexpectedly, the latter two components emerged as a greater focus of concern within this category than did independence or self-reliance. For instance:

> #147: I'd like them to be productive and creative. That we encourage them to use all their mental facilities. That they just not take things for granted. . . . That they not only be productive and creative and feel good about themselves, but that they project that towards something they can do for the rest of their lives.

> #164: I hope he's just happy. . . . Umm, you know, goes to school, learns a good, you know, good trade or something so he can get out there and get ahead in life. That's what I want, I want him to, you know—have a goal in life. Make goals and reach for them.

A few mothers elaborated at length on the quality of independence in and of itself, but generally independence or self-reliance was either secondary to or embedded within what appeared to be the more central goals of "feeling good about yourself" and "striving to be all you can be":

> #148: I don't really want them to limit themselves. I want them to feel like the world is their oyster, and it's there for them. . . . I want them to be—to accept themselves the way they are, just be happy the way they are, and do things by themselves, and find a thing they enjoy doing and put their whole heart into it. . . . I'd like them to be individuals, to think for themselves. I want them to be confident.

> #151: I guess the main thing is to feel good about themselves and to be self-assured. . . . And, you know, I think everything else falls into place if they feel good about themselves.

> #154: The first thing that comes to mind would be a good sense of self-esteem. To me, that seems to be the key to every other thing that you do in life. And I guess the next that I would think of would be independence.

This emphasis was not limited to adult socialization goals. It was not unusual for mothers to describe 12-month-olds in terms of their capacity for self-enhancement, happiness, and self-reliance:

> #150: She's, uh, always been a very self-contained child. She has a lot of inner resources. She's able to calm herself. She takes a lot of joy in her surroundings.

> #148: And she's a very intelligent child . . . and she's always smiling, and she likes to think and—she's just a little baby . . . [but] she likes to see how things go together. She's just a happy baby, and I admire her because she just—she's in a day care environment, and she makes the best of the situation, and she learns from everything that she does. She's just a happy baby, you know.

Significantly, even the domain of emotional connectedness to others—a quality coded under the Lovingness category—frequently appeared in mothers' interviews as one inner capacity among many that are key to the development of one's full potential as a human being and concomitant subjective satisfaction:

#142: Well, I would like my child or future children to feel, uh, secure and to take time to enjoy life, to enjoy relationships with other people. To be curious about the world. To have an idea of what their own special gifts are and to develop them as much as possible. To have a sort of enthusiasm about life.

#146: To learn everything that he can possibly learn, go to college. I guess just to be a happy person. Enjoy life. . . . Friendly, outgoing, happy, active, he loves people, he loves to play, he loves to read, he loves to experience new things.

More broadly, emotions themselves—or at least how they are dealt with—were treated as an index of one's self-development: The fully realized human being should be able to identify feelings, express them when it is appropriate to do so, and control them when it is not. The proper regulation of feelings and needs was viewed as indicative of one's ability to cope, and thus of one's self-development, happiness, and autonomy:

#147: That they can help identify what it is that they're feeling and thinking, and be able to do something about it—to help themselves. I'd like all of that toward them doing something with their lives that they feel happy with.

#151: She's very articulate and she's at ease with others. She can easily say what she's feeling and talk about things because she feels good about herself. And I think that maybe the ability to communicate and to relate to others is something that comes from this self-assurance and this internal happiness.

Thus, across socioeconomic status, the Anglo mothers in this study expressed substantial concern that their children develop the skills and abilities to "get ahead in life," to be able not only to "make it" but to "make it on their own," and to experience a sense of subjective satisfaction in the process. These combined emphases on autonomy, satisfaction with one's self and one's life, and the development of skills and abilities—which we together called Self-Maximization—represented on average 65% of each middle-class and 51% of each working-class Anglo mother's responses to the question, "What qualities would you like your child to come to possess as he/she grows older?"

EMOTIONS AND SELF-MAXIMIZATION

As mentioned earlier, a counterpoint to the concern with Self-Maximiztion was substantial consideration of the place of emotions. Emotions were generally viewed either as negatively interfering with the process of Self-Maximization, or as indicative of its attainment. There were two primary ways in which emotions appeared to be an index of Self-Maximization: (1) The ability to identify, understand, and appropriately express one's feelings was regarded as an important component of self-awareness and a skill that would allow an individual to "get your needs met" and so "get more out of life"; and (2) the capacity for love, empathy, and emotional connectedness to others was judged crucial to happiness, inasmuch as it counteracts the ultimate aloneness each of us must confront as autonomous individuals.

Expressing Yourself and Getting Your Needs Met

Emotions were described by many mothers as indicators of internal needs, wants, and desires. The ability to identify and appropriately express these needs was viewed as key to satisfying them:

> #146: He has his own little personality. He knows how to get attention from people; he knows how to get his needs met.

> #147: I'd like for them to in some ways to be able to think clearly through how *they* feel about things and that they can work out problems, and that they could be at peace with themselves and be really secure.

> #166: She's got her own personality; she knows what she likes, what she doesn't like. She basically does things on her own. . . . She's only, what, 18 months and she can repeat words like you wouldn't believe. . . . She knows words. You know, so—I mean, she can basically tell you what's wrong with her. And to me that's a very good [quality].

Emotions were thus viewed as a part of oneself, and knowing how to identify and appropriately express them was seen as crucial to self-awareness and autonomy. Implicit within this formulation is the belief that individuals are responsible for letting others know what they feel; persons who can articulate their needs are more likely to get those needs met than persons who cannot.

Emotional Connectedness to Others

A major theme for the Anglo mothers was concern that their children develop the capacity for emotional connectedness to others. Relatedness to others was viewed both as an ability within a child and as a potential source of subjective satisfaction—a part of the world that is there for the child to enjoy. The failure to be able to find joy in relationships was viewed as a limitation on the ability to self-maximize:

> #142: . . . to feel, uh, secure and to take time to enjoy life, to enjoy relationships with other people. . . . You don't want him or her to feel paranoid about how other people feel about them. To have a fairly optimistic opinion about the possibilities for relationships with other people.

> #155: I would like them to be happy and satisfied in their jobs, and just to be able to enjoy a lot of variety of things. So the emotional ones are mainly that they're happy with their life, and, umm, that they are able to know how to enjoy a wide variety of things and people.

> #164: He's an actor. He can put on a show. He can make you laugh so hard. He's funny. He's got a good personality already. It's already coming out. I think he—he already makes friends. . . . I think he'll have a lot of friends.

The Anglo mothers, then, viewed the capacity for relatedness as an internal ability, a source of potential satisfaction, and an index of a general enthusiasm and joy in living. As they saw it, a person who lacks the ability to relate to others is likely also to be a person who is isolated and unhappy:

> #142: I can think of a girl who's in his playgroup who never smiles. . . . She was very advanced in a lot of ways for her age, but she didn't seem to have much pleasure in life, and she didn't seem to have any interest in other kids, except as obstacles.

> #146: And he's very quiet, didn't talk at an early age, somewhat autistic, beginning to be verbal. . . . But not very social. Doesn't smile much. Doesn't laugh much. . . . I'd hate to see [my child] distrust people, dislike people. . . . I'd hate to have a child who was miserable.

> #170: She's really, really shy. She don't talk or nothing like that, at least not with people she don't know . . . it's like she has no personality except for the people who she's closest with.

Despite its importance, emotional connectedness was also presented as potentially in tension with Self-Maximization. That is, if the child being described was viewed as lacking sufficient autonomy, then the positive desire for emotional closeness and nurturing turned instead into a negative dependence:

> #143: I really don't enjoy seeing little kids who are totally clingy and dependent on the parents. Who, even though they know you well and know your house, just won't move from their mother's lap to play. I'd like them to be somewhat independent.

> #157: We're very lucky. He's not a very clingy child. So he's not clingy with me, and he's not clingy with his day care mother, although he loves being at day care with her. But he doesn't need to be, you know, coddled all the time, which is great.

> #174: But like I said, she's a real happy-go-lucky kid, and she's not one of those whiny kids that hang on you all the time.

As the Anglo mothers viewed it, then, relatedness is something that must be tempered with—and, ideally, grows out of—a strong sense of self.

Balance of Autonomy and Relatedness

For the Anglo mothers, both autonomy and relatedness thus appeared to be necessary qualities for self-development. If positive emotional connectedness was absent, then the child being described was portrayed as emotionally isolated, barren, or unhappy. On the other hand, a child who lacked autonomy was depicted as clingy, dependent, and unable to stand on his or her own two feet. What was seen as most desirable, then, was finding an optimal balance between autonomy and relatedness—a balance that was frequently viewed as part of reaching one's full potential:

> #143: [She's] not afraid to climb on her mother's lap, but also very able to play by herself.

> #146: I'd like him to be independent and love us, but stand on his own.

> #174: Not to grow up with a—kinda attitude that she doesn't need anybody. You know. That friends are good to have. . . .

Yeah, you know, I want her to be independent, but yet, you know, it's good to have other people around to be with and stuff.

#261: Just to have a mind of their own and not be talked into something else; I was in a job for 5 years that I hated because I listened to my father. With my 10-year-old, I'd like her to be more selfish; she does too much for others. I'd like her to do for others, but not so much that it takes away from her.

For the Anglo mothers, then, autonomy and emotional connectedness appeared to be opposite ends of a teeter-totter seeking a weighted balance. Too little autonomy, and the child would be enmeshed in overdependence, trapped in an ill-defined sense of self, or turned into a doormat for others; too much autonomy, and the child would be emotionally isolated and barren, cut off from the world and unable to enjoy life. From this perspective, the individual lives among others, but is necessarily separate from them. Psychological health requires knowing how to balance and resolve this fundamental tension between self and other.

EMOTIONS AND SELF-MAXIMIZATION IN TENSION

As described above, the abilities to express one's needs and to have meaningful emotional connections were viewed as essential to Self-Maximization. However, there also emerged in these interviews a picture of emotions as potentially dangerous forces that require proper control and regulation, lest they hinder the attainment of one's goals, the capacity for self-reliance, or the search for happiness. There were three primary emotional dimensions or tendencies within the individual, the proper regulation of which was considered requisite to Self-Maximization: (1) anger, including aggression and the ability to tolerate frustration; (2) selfishness or greed; and (3) egocentrism or intolerance.

Anger

Anger, including aggression and the inability to tolerate frustration, emerged as a major theme in Anglo mothers' descriptions of what they would not like to see in their own children. Often, anger and aggression were described as occurring in response to frustration of a child's desires:

#162: He's already got a temper, so I'd like him to be able to control his temper to a certain degree, you know. You ask him to do something, if he doesn't want to do it, it's—"No," or "Wahh," start screaming.

#173: [She] doesn't like to be told what to do. Screams, yells, throws tantrums whenever she can't get her own way.

The regulation of anger was considered a necessary ability. For some mothers, aggression appeared to be linked with problematic behavior that could interfere with the achievement of other positive life goals:

#164: Well, he already has this thing with hitting and punching. I hope he doesn't become a troublemaker. . . . I want him to have a good perspective on life, you know. . . . [What do you mean by a good perspective?] You know, I don't want him to—it's hard to explain—to think that hanging out is cool, and doing drugs is cool, and getting in fights is cool, just to be popular or something, because it's not. It's really stupid, and you only end up getting in trouble.

The inability to cope with frustration was also considered to be indicative of poor coping skills, thus undermining potential self-control and autonomy:

#151: He's incredibly, umm, easily frustrated, and every little thing sort of sets him off. Well, he used to bang his head. He'd get so frustrated about something, you know, that he'd bang his—he just couldn't handle it. He just couldn't cope with, like, not being able to put a puzzle piece in. He'd sort of throw the puzzle piece across the floor, throw himself on the floor, and bang his head. . . . Because I think that would be a horrible cross to bear through life. Everything is just huge balls of frustration at every turn.

#156: And so, umm, just not being a hothead, blow up easy about things, have a tantrum—to be more—being able to cool off and think about things and be a little more rational.

At times, the need to control anger was considered to be in conflict with the ability to be open and self-expressive:

#157: I want him to be open with his emotions, but first of all there's a big difference between allowing him to feel, for instance, mad at me and hitting me, and knowing that hitting me's not a good thing. . . . So I don't—in order to know that his emotions are all right, but that he needs to be able to curb certain ones.

Finally, anger's undesirability was attributed partly to the fact that it mitigates against the ability to enjoy life:

#154: He's an angry child—he's always hitting out on other kids. He has an unhappy look.

#147: That they not be so stressed out and uptight about themselves and everything else that they can't be happy.

In sum, the capacity to tolerate frustration was considered crucial; the Anglo mothers believed that a lack of this ability could hinder the achievement of positive life goals, undermine self-control and autonomy, interfere with appropriate self-expressiveness, and leave one unhappy. The proper control of anger and aggression was thus considered requisite to Self-Maximization.

Selfishness and Egocentrism

Selfishness and egocentrism surfaced as two other very common concerns among the Anglo mothers. Often, the inability to share was viewed as a correlate of aggressiveness and low frustration tolerance, and was considered to limit one's capacity to enjoy life and to cope with life's minor adversities:

#142: I can think of a girl who's in his playgroup who never smiles. . . . She's also very selfish and pushy with other kids. She'd actually go up and scratch one of the kids or just sort of attack them . . . she didn't seem to have much pleasure in life, and she didn't seem to have any interest in other kids, except as obstacles.

#148: [This child] used to go to my sister's day care, who used to fight with all the little babies; he used to fight with the children, and he was very selfish. And he used to scream all the time . . . he was just a very unhappy child.

#173: Selfish, yeah. Very selfish. Doesn't like to be told what to do. Screams, yells, throws tantrums whenever she can't get her own way. Hits.

At other times, selfishness was interpreted more broadly as an inability to extend oneself—an excess of individualism that transformed positive autonomy into negative egocentrism and consequent emotional isolation:

> #144: Manipulative, self-centered. Very much into her own world. Doesn't share with other children.

> #151: I think that certainly self-centeredness I think is good to a certain degree, but I wouldn't want a child to be so selfish that he, you know, sort of expects of others. I'd like him to have friends, you know, to be able to make friends.

> #162: I wouldn't want him to be nasty, or a pushy type of person, or, uh, you know, to demand a lot, or stuff like that. You know, I wouldn't want him to think he has control over everything, and you know, "*I* come first," or this or that.

From this perspective, emotions are not only potentially dangerous forces within a person that need to be regulated; they can also be the negative consequences of an excessive individualism. A person who cares *only* about himself or herself will be aggressive, selfish, egocentric, and ultimately friendless. The desire and the capacity to relate to others thus temper an unrestrained ego. Here again, balance is key.

PERCEPTIONS OF ATTACHMENT BEHAVIOR

A balance between autonomy and relatedness was a major theme in Study 2 Anglo mothers' perceptions of the two hypothetical toddlers whose behavior they generally found most desirable (Lee and Kelly, the "distal" B1 and B2 toddlers; see the Appendix) in a simulated Strange Situation. This was true across socioeconomic class:

> #249: Because I like his being comfortable left alone and self-confident, but is interested in relationships and relating to others.

> #251: Content, well-adjusted, confident. Good relationship with his mother, but gets along on his own when he has to.

> #276: To be secure with himself and his surroundings, but noticed his mother was gone—aware of her absence, but didn't totally distress him because he felt safe; played nicely, happy, well balanced.

#277: Adjusted—what I would expect a toddler to do; in tune with his mom, but he could play by himself; concerned she was leaving, but didn't feel he was being abandoned; when she came back, it was just a little reassurance he wanted.

Anglo mothers' perceptions of desirable Strange Situation behavior thus corresponded closely to their descriptions of qualities they would like their children to possess. Optimal Strange Situation behavior involved a balance between a healthy autonomy and a capacity for relatedness. The toddler who demonstrated both of these qualities in the Strange Situation was considered "well adjusted."

Similarly, mothers' perceptions of undesirable Strange Situation behavior coincided with their characterizations of qualities they would not like their children to possess. For instance, the highly avoidant (A1) toddler, Alex, was praised for independence but criticized for emotional detachment:

#242: Independent, curious, active, not attached to her mother much for that age, rambunctious . . . would want her to play independently, but would like her to acknowledge that I left and returned.

#253: Was able to play and use his imagination, but doesn't seem very interested in people.

#278: Not very alert to her mother—interested in the toys, but not alert to what's going on around her, not too attached to her mother.

#262: Into herself—doesn't care about anything; into playing with her toys.

On the other hand, the "clingy" (proximal) B4 toddler, Chris, was criticized for being overly dependent but appreciated for caring about the mother:

#241: It's nice to be wanted—mine never cries when I leave her; but I wouldn't want her to be too clingy—I'll come back and she need not fear that [I won't].

#250: There's something a little gratifying in your child's dependency and attachment—you feel needed, know he looks to you; but at the same time, it's good to know he can be independent for a while and can understand you'll be back and that this is a safe environment.

#269: Because you never want your child to be crying, but you also like that they love you so much they can't be out of your sight.

#274: Because I'd want my kids to feel attached to me, count on me, but would like them not to be upset if I leave—to feel reassured and not have to cry; be used to the fact that sometimes I'll have to leave.

Finally, Anglo mothers felt that the extremely clingy, angry C1 toddler, Lindsay, lacked the capacity to regulate his or her emotions, responding to frustration of his or her wishes with anger. This failure to self-regulate was perceived to portend an inability to cope with life's minor adversities, and thus a lack of autonomy or self-confidence:

#245: Expressing anger; seemed unsure of what she wanted, unsure of herself. . . . I want to be able to go into a new situation and feel confident she'll be able to adjust to a new environment.

#253: Seems frustrated; mad at his mom for leaving; not able to control his emotions by sucking his thumb and crying. Wouldn't want him to get upset that easily; would want him to be able to get over his upset a little more quickly.

#272: Spoiled; probably gets a lot of attention and everything his own way, and every time he cries he probably gets his way. Won't get too far in life, because he's going to find out you don't get everything you want.

#279: Insecure with her mother leaving; figures that because her mother left her, she would fight back, rebel, when she returns. Like, "You did this to me, so I'm going to do it back to you." It's like they want to crawl back inside you, be with them always. But they need to learn to be on their own, because I don't want them to feel that insecure, to be so dependent on me.

In sum, there was considerable concordance between mothers' descriptions of qualities they would and would not like their own children to possess, and their perceptions of desirable and undesirable Strange Situation behavior. In particular, both middle- and working-class Anglo mothers emphasized the importance of an optimal balance between autonomy and relatedness. Desirable Strange Situation behavior consisted of displaying sufficient autonomy to explore the toys and to cope with a brief separation, yet at the same time demonstrating enough relatedness to miss the mother while she was gone and to be happy when she returned. Undesirable Strange Situation behavior included imbalances in the autonomy–relatedness continuum, such that a toddler seemed either emotionally detached or too dependent. However, an inability to regulate anger and frustration was also perceived to be undesirable, inasmuch as it indicated an incapacity to cope with minor adversities, and thus a lack of optimal self-development. This conceptualizaton of Strange Situation behavior maps well onto the traditional conceptualization of Group B behavior as representing an optimal balance in the child's ability to explore independently and to relate to others.

This conceptualization of Strange Situation behavior is also consistent with a depiction of dominant U.S. culture as individualistic. In this view, the self represents "a dynamic center of awareness, emotion, judgment and action organized into a distinctive whole and set contrastively both against other such wholes and against its social and natural background" (Geertz, 1984, p. 126). Or, as Kessen (1979, p. 819) puts it, "The child . . . is invariably seen as a . . . self-contained and complete individual." He or she is influenced, to be sure, by "other similarly self-contained people," but ultimately it is the child who is "the container of self and of psychology. Impulses are in the child; traits are in the child; thoughts are in the child; attachments are in the child." U.S. discourse thus introduces a basic dualism between self and other; one's responsibility to others is frequently perceived to be in tension with one's responsibility to self (Cushman, 1991). The capacity to resolve this tension—to find a satisfactory balance between autonomy and relatedness—is key to optimal personal health.

A similar dualism dominates U.S. discourse on emotion. As Lutz (1990, p. 69) notes, "Another and competing theme in Western cultural renditions of emotion . . . contrasts emotion with cold alienation. Emotion, in this view, is life to its absence's death, is interpersonal connection or relationship to an unemotional estrangement, is a glorified and free nature against a shackling civilization." Emotion is also "irrational rather than rational, chaotic rather than ordered . . . unintended and uncontrollable, and hence often dangerous." In short, emotions are a force welling up within the self that can either provide warmth and so counteract the ultimate aloneness each individual must face, or wreak havoc on a person's inner capacity to meet adversity with confidence, resourcefulness, and equanimity. In this way, emotions can either enhance the self or hinder it in its search for inner completion.

In keeping with this perspective, when asked to appraise the behavior of the C1 toddler in a simulated Strange Situation, Anglo mothers divided 68% (working-class) and 80% (middle-class) of their total number of responses between the Self-Maximization and Self-Control categories. For all other toddlers, Anglo mothers distributed 61–80% (working-class) and 83–92% (middle-class) of their total number of responses between the Self-Maximization and Lovingness categories. As is evident, these tendencies were more marked among the middle-class mothers, but were nonetheless strong for the working-class mothers as well.

CHAPTER FIVE

Images of the Child:
Respect and Affection

◆

Just as it has become increasingly common to point to the individualism of dominant U.S. culture, it has also become customary to contrast this individualism with an alternative mode of ordering the relations between self and other. Following Shweder and Bourne (1984), we have chosen to call this perspective "sociocentric," but it has also been variously termed, among other things, "interdependent," "holistic," "collective," and "allocentric" (Marin & Triandis, 1985; Markus & Kitayama, 1991). Basically, in this perspective, the self is assumed to be an integral part of the social context rather than an autonomous unit moving within it. For instance, Markus and Kitayama (1991) contrast the internal, private features of the "independent" self, whose goal is to be unique and expressive, with the external, public roles of the "interdependent" self, whose aim is to belong and to maintain harmony. Although this general contrast between individualistic and sociocentric meaning systems is a useful heuristic device, most researchers agree that individualism and sociocentrism will have different contours in different sociocultural groups (Markus & Kitayama, 1991). For instance, Japanese, Chinese, and Hindu cultures can all be described as "sociocentric," just as U.S. and German cultures can both be called "individualistic." However, few people would argue that all Asian cultures are identical, any more than they would contend that all Western ones are—or even that cultures themselves are homogeneous units, devoid of within-group variability. In this book, we are interested in going beyond a general characterization of individualistic versus sociocentric cultures to more in-depth analyses of the perceptions of middle- and working-class Anglo and Puerto Rican mothers. As in Chapter Four, we focus in this chapter on within-group commonalities, this time among the Puerto Rican mothers. We discuss within-group differences in Chapter Six.

PROPER DEMEANOR

Whereas the overriding concern of the Anglo mothers in our studies was to promote in their children an optimal balance of autonomy and relatedness, the Puerto Rican mothers focused primarily on the ability of their children to engage in contextually appropriate levels of relatedness. Chief among these levels is a dimension of behavior that we called Proper Demeanor. Although Proper Demeanor implicitly assumes appropriate relatedness (both intimate and nonintimate), it also assumes a quality that is perhaps best described in English as "teachable" and in Spanish as *educado*. The child who is *educado* (well taught, well brought up), as opposed to *malcriado* (poorly taught, poorly brought up), is one who is *tranquilo, obediente,* and *respetuoso.* That is, the child is calm, obedient, and respectfully attentive to the teachings of his or her elders, in order to become skilled in the interpersonal and rhetorical competencies that will someday be expected of the well-socialized adult (C. L. Briggs, 1986; Diaz Royo, 1974; Lucca, 1988).

Respeto

Proper Demeanor is intrinsically contextual; it involves, by definition, knowing the level of courtesy and decorum required in a given situation in relation to other people of a particular age, sex, and social status. The cardinal rule governing Proper Demeanor in Puerto Rico is *respeto,* or respect, which will manifest itself differently in different contexts (Lauria, 1982). As one middle-class Puerto Rican mother described it:

> #02: I would love it if they were . . . *respetuosos* (respectful) toward their elders as well as with people their own age, so that when they're adolescents and then adults, they know how to use particular aspects of their personality at the appropriate time, so that others will *respetan* (respect) them.

Although intrinsically contextual, this mother's final comment suggests a second crucial dimension of *respeto*: It is public. The ability to maintain *respeto* defines who you are as a person and how others will respond to you. The positive evaluation of others is prerequisite to good standing in the community and necessary to survival. The person who lacks the ability to maintain *respeto* is *un malcriado*—one who has been poorly brought up.

> #38: Perhaps that is one of the reasons I would not like [my child to be *malcriado*]—because he would end up feeling rejected, including feeling others' harsh looks because he is like that. Nobody wants to take care of a *malcriado* child; nobody wants to be with him.

> #27: People more highly value children who *respetan* their elders; they admire them more. And even though sometimes it is hard for me [to instill *respeto* in my children], it is one of the most important things.

> #04: A child who is not *respetuoso* will not become anything; nobody will like them, everyone will turn them away, they will speak poorly of him.

Also apparent in these passages is the extent to which, for the Puerto Rican mothers, one's life is lived under the watchful eyes of an observing community that has the power to offer either love and acceptance or rejection and pain. The esteem of the community is paramount, and such esteem is granted only when one comports oneself with *respeto*.

Obediente, Tranquilo, and Amable

As suggested earlier, the demands of Proper Demeanor vary with age, gender, and social status. For all children in Puerto Rico, it includes being *obediente* (obedient), *tranquilo* (calm), and *amable* (polite, gentle, kind). A child who is *intranquilo* (restless) lacks the capacity to attend to others' needs and wishes, and a child who is disobedient or impolite defies authority. Such children are *malcriados,* a term that can be translated not only as "poorly brought up" but also as "ill-mannered."

> #08: I cannot stand *irrespetuosos* (disrespectful children) or *malcriados*.

#17: I know some children who are *malcriados,* who lack *respeto* for older people.

#58: I would like him to be *respetuoso*, that he would not be *irrespetuoso*—hmm, that he would not be a bad son, that he would not be mean to others, that he would be unhelpful, that he would not be *malcriado*.

In a young child, being *obediente* in particular is an essential component of *respeto*. A child who is disobedient by definition challenges the authority of his or her elders, thus behaving disrespectfully:

#04: I don't like it when I send him to do something and he tells me no, because that makes me mad, it infuriates me; he should *respetar* what I say. What other person will he say that to when they ask him to do something? He will simply stay there as if nothing were going on; he will keep singing or walking along. I know this, because sometimes I tell him, "Look at me," and he keeps doing what he was doing as if I were not there. . . . I knew a boy, my nephew, who is not here right now. He was *respetuoso*; one sent him to do something and he did it quietly, without talking back or anything like that.

#17: You know that when you scold her, well, she is going to listen; I tell her, "Look, you do not touch that," and, well, she does not touch it. . . . In this I refer to *respeto*. One tells her, "No, no, you cannot touch that," and she won't touch it. "Don't pick that up, don't put that in your mouth, well, give it to me," and she does. When she takes something—a penny or something—to put in her mouth, and I say, "No, nasty, give me," and I put out my hand and she gives it to me, well, there is *respeto*, and for her age she understands.

#03: [There is] a girl I know who is the same age as mine, 1 year and 9 months. This little girl is *obediente*, even though she is so young, *respeta* her mother and things like that. Well, [she is] *obediente* because every time the mother tells her to come and sit down here, she comes, eats her food and everything. . . . [I wouldn't like my child to be] *desobediente,* because if one has always taught him to *respetar* his elders and those who are around him, and to *obedecer* (obey) what one tells him to do, then he should be *obediente*.

A child also demonstrates *respeto* through behavior that is *tranquilo* (calm). Children who are *tranquilos* possess the necessary capacity to be attentive to others on at least three different levels. Children who are *intranquilos* will be (1) bothersome to other adults; (2) immodestly calling undue attention to themselves through noise and activity, thus embarrassing themselves and their families; and (3) unable to be attentive and therefore obedient to their elders:

> #08: She cannot remain still next to her mother. She calls a lot of attention to herself; they cannot place her in a playpen and have her remain *tranquila*.

> #13: She knows how to behave. She goes to other people's homes, sits down, and is very *tranquila* and *respetuosa*. She doesn't bother anyone, and I enjoy taking care of her. . . . [I know a girl who] is 1 year and 5 months. [She] is very naughty. When you call her, she doesn't listen. She isn't *tranquila*; she's always running, never *tranquila*, and very mischievous.

> #34: Well, that boy is a *tranquilo* boy. He likes to play but he isn't very *intranquilo*; he is an *obediente* boy, he listens to his parents.

Finally, a child also manifests *respeto* through behavior that is *amable*. A term that is difficult to translate into English, *amable* is a blend of politeness, gentleness, kindness, and goodness. *Amable* is used to describe an attitude one presents in interactions with others, as well as behaviors communicating that attitude. It is a quality of positive relatedness, but one that is shown to all people, not just friends and other intimates, and thus belongs to the domain of Proper Demeanor:

> #30: I don't like a child who is *malcriado*, who acts like he is *malcriado* in front of anyone, wants everything he sees; he doesn't know when they tell him no, they have to buy him everything. And he isn't even *amable*; he isn't even sociable with people [he meets] in the street. He isn't *amable*, and he makes his mother look bad.

> #46: I would like for my son to be *respetuoso*, *amable*, *obediente*. I would like him to be that way so that one does not have to have a hard time [dealing] with the boy.

> #25: Who doesn't wish the best for their child? I would like for mine the best qualities in the world—that he would be *cariñoso* (affectionate), *respetuoso*, responsible, *amable*, good, and intelligent. I want these qualities because I love him. He's my son. I want him to be a good child.

In sum, a Puerto Rican child who is *educado* is one who is *respetuoso*, and the way in which a child demonstrates *respeto* is through behavior that is *obediente* to elders, *tranquilo* enough to attend to others' needs, and *amable* to all. The child who behaves in these culturally prescribed ways will gain the esteem and affection of the larger community, whereas the child who does not will be spurned. These findings are consonant with those of Lucca (1988), who concludes that her sample of children from a Puerto Rican fishing village were more likely than U.S. mainland children to construe themselves through the positive or negative reactions that their behaviors elicited from others. For example, when asked to describe what was most important about themselves, Puerto Rican children were likely to answer in a way that was extremely uncommon among U.S. children: "[It is most important to] be nice and respect people. . . . Because if I'm bad everybody will hit and hate me. When I would be in danger they would not help me" (quoted in Lucca, 1988, p. 164).

Puerto Rican children thus learn that if they lack Proper Demeanor they will find themselves outcasts, alone, and unable to survive. Proper Demeanor and its cardinal principle, *respeto,* are therefore crucial to a child's happiness and well-being. Proper Demeanor is also an intrinsically public quality; it is played out in the arena of interpersonal relationships, both intimate and nonintimate. It inevitably immerses an individual in a complex web of expectations and obligations, the successful negotiation of which will require obedience in childhood, and polite attentiveness throughout life.

Vergüenza

Proper Demeanor is more than a set of behaviors. It also entails a dimension of feeling known as *vergüenza* or "shame." The person who possesses the capacity to feel *vergüenza* is able to take responsibility for his or her behavior. Ideally, the *educado* Puerto Rican adult is always a person *de vergüenza*—that is, continually conscious of the potential for shame through loss of face in any interpersonal setting (Crespo, 1986; Diaz Royo, 1974). A lack of sense of *vergüenza* increases the possibility that one will breach expectations of proper demeanor and thus suffer shame. However, *vergüenza* is not only something one feels as a result of one's own misdeeds; it is also something one experiences because of the misconduct of family members.

Thus, children who behave poorly shame not only themselves, but also their parents, who have failed to rear them properly:

> #49: [I wouldn't like my child to] be bothersome, *malcriado*, or *irrespetuoso*. I do not like children who are bothersome, because then they raise Cain and they do not *respetan* others; thereafter people begin to say that you do not teach your children *vergüenza*.

> #55: [When this child comes into a public place], he gets excited and trips over all the furniture, throws the toys, and does not listen to anyone. He does this because he is *malcriado* and his parents do not teach him *vergüenza*.

> #46: [I will] make sure that [my son] is not *malcriado*, nosy, or a liar, because the worst thing in the world is a *malcriado* boy, you know—the *vergüenza* they make you go through.

For Puerto Rican children, then, breaches of Proper Demeanor have negative consequences not only for themselves, but also for their families. Inasmuch as families or parents are responsible for teaching children the ways of *respeto*, an individual's lack thereof reflects poorly on the family as a whole. To be continually conscious in any interaction of the potential for *vergüenza* through loss of face is prerequisite to being a truly moral person—one who guards not only his or her own honor, but that of the family as well.

UNA PERSONA DE PROVECHO

A person who fulfills the requirements of *respeto* and lives a life of honor is *una persona de provecho*, a person who is worthy of trust and useful to society. *Provecho* encompasses a set of characteristics generally subsumed in English under the rubric of "integrity" or "decency": *Una persona de provecho* is responsible, honest, hard-working, morally upright, and God-fearing, and accepts the consequences of his or her own actions. In Puerto Rico, however, these qualities are viewed less as internalized principles of right and wrong, and more as the cohesive glue of society. *De provecho* has connotations not only of moral goodness, but of societal usefulness as well: *Una persona de provecho* can be trusted to fulfill his or her obligations (whatever they may be) to family, friends, neighbors, coworkers, and the community as a whole. Such a person is fully human in the deepest sense, and gains the regard of others:

> #09: Well, I'd like them to be *personas de provecho* in the future, that they'd be *tranquilo,* uh, people who are well known, others know them, people well loved in their community and by others. . . . They need to have *provecho.* . . . I'd like them to be sociable, to share, be in a club, one of those clubs so they could help others, be attentive—not just be people who let life go by. I'd like them to help their community.

The process of becoming *una persona de provecho* is lifelong, and must begin in early childhood. Children must be taught the necessary virtues if they are to become *personas de provecho* and thus gain honor and affection in the eyes of the observing community:

> #45: That she be *una nena hogareña, de su casa* [literally, "a girl of her home, of her house"—one who does not wander the streets, but protects her reputation and fulfills her obligations as a daughter], responsible, and serious. I would like her to be this way so that in the future she will receive *respeto* from other people. . . . Quiet, responsible, serious, *educada.* That she makes other people like her.

> #56: Well, I'd like him to be *cariñoso, obediente,* playful, not too active, excessively active. I'd like him to be honest—that is, to tell the truth. Faithful to his parents. . . . Because I understand that these are the qualities that you can teach them from the time they're small; then little by little as they grow up, if they have these same virtues, then they can do good, be a good human being when they're grown.

> #11: I would like him to be very honest, very responsible. But responsible not only in the sense of being punctual, which is a part of responsibility, but also responsible for his actions. When he commits an—an act which is wrong, that he knows how to face it, and he knows how to—hmmm—accept, you know, to say, "I did this wrong, let me see how I can fix this," and that he also be responsible for himself, you know, for his clothes; if he throws them down that he picks them up, and for his toys. Because now he is at a stage where he is learning to play and to socialize with other children, and I would like him to be, you know, responsible for himself, for everything he does . . . that he knows how to conduct himself.

In this way, qualities of integrity are viewed as intrinsically social. A child who is responsible is one who "knows how to conduct himself" or herself, and such a child will "do good" and be respected by others when he or she is grown.

PROPER DEMEANOR AND THE EMOTIONS

Concern for both positive and negative emotions emerged among the Puerto Rican mothers in our research, as it did for the Anglo mothers. However, rather than being viewed as forces that can enhance the self or hinder its completion, emotions were depicted by the Puerto Rican mothers instead as resulting in behaviors that can either strengthen or threaten the regard and well-being of others in the community.

Cariño and Confianza

Like the Anglo mothers, the Puerto Rican mothers interviewed in these studies wanted their children to have warm, affectionate relationships with others. However, the Anglo mothers tended to see relationships as potentially in tension with and optimally balancing the goal of Self-Maximization. In their view, relationships are commodities that can alleviate one's sense of aloneness and lend greater joy to one's life, but they can also imperil independence and so must be tempered with autonomy. The Puerto Rican mothers, on the other hand, appeared to consider emotional connectedness and Proper Demeanor as distinct but interdependent; being *cariñoso* (affectionate, sweet) is a quality of warmth that, together with *respeto*, is essential to gaining the esteem and love of others. If *respeto* defines the intricate courtesies and obligations that are requisite to negotiating the social world, then *cariño* (affection) can sweeten this negotiation with warmth and love. Together, *respeto* and *cariño* define different levels of acceptance by the community. The child who is *respetuoso* gains the approval of the community by displaying the social decorum necessary in all interactions; the child who is *cariñoso* as well as *respetuoso* elicits love and admiration:

> #02: [My daughter is] very courteous, very *cariñosa*, very friendly. No matter where I go with her—to the market, to the movies, or to eat at a restaurant—she gets everyone's attention, she touches

everyone's heart. That is when I notice how loving she is. She touches people when she gets close to them; immediately she breaks that person's heart, because that person, well, immediately gives her attention, carries her, or attempts to kiss her, touch her, because she is so *cariñosa* and courteous with them.

#56: To me, he's a wonderful boy. It's not because he's my son, but because he's very *cariñoso*, he's expressive, he's loving in terms of touching; he expresses love with words and with touch; he's sincere. He's faithful with everyone . . . and that is beautiful, because he makes everyone love him.

#27: I like them to express the *cariño* they have toward me, toward others. I believe *cariñoso* children make you love them more than children who are more independent.

#24: Well, for example, my son is barely 18 months old, and he is very *cariñoso* and at the same time very demonstrative. He is one of those to whom the whole world says, "I love you," and he kisses the whole world, and at only 18 months; I consider that a highly advanced stage, for he knows that in giving love he receives love.

An additional level of belonging is denoted by the term *confianza* (trust). *Confianza* exists between intimates, and helps to define one's closest relationships. *Confianza* is also a specific characteristic of the mother–child relationships; it allows the child to be open to the mother's attempts to *educar* the child (bring him or her up properly):

#17: [I hope] that she has a good example from me as a mother. . . . Whatever I could offer, you know, the love and everything that I could offer to her, well, when she has her own children, well, she can develop it in them as well; she can do the same things with her own children. Offer them love, *respeto*, confidence, and *confianza*. I hope that [my daughter] will *confíe* (confide) in me a lot. . . . I would talk a lot with her, not like a mother—you know, but like a friend that she *confíe* (confides in). And then, having her *confianza* in me, well, then I would tell her, "Well, look, I would not like for you to do such and such, because I went through this, this, and this."

#30: I believe, to start, that if they don't lie and are sincere and honest, and if they have *confianza* in me, this—they are going to, going to be growing closer to me, and they will tell me what they do, and what their worries are. And in this way I can be more in control of the path that they are taking in life, and in this way also I think they will become men of good, and it would be harder for them to become sidetracked into drugs or quitting school and things like that.

#10: One needs to understand [children when they misbehave], because they like to do things their way. If they are going to make it in life, one must give them *confianza*, and when you give them this *confianza*, then you can find a way to strive together.

For the Puerto Rican mothers, then, relatedness is not in tension with Self-Maximization, as it is among the Anglo mothers, but is instead its multilayered expression. In this view, the self finds fulfillment only with acceptance by the community, and such acceptance comes as a result of the successful negotiation of social relationships at multiple levels, beginning with the *confianza*, *cariño*, and *respeto* that exist between parents and children. From this perspective, proper relatedness, not bounded but sociable separateness, is the highest goal of the individual and the endpoint of development.

Aggression, Greed, and Egotism

Like the Anglo mothers, Puerto Rican mothers expressed concern that their children learn to control negative tendencies toward aggression, greed, and egotism. However, whereas Anglo mothers tended to focus on these as factors hindering Self-Maximization, Puerto Rican mothers appeared to view them as drives giving rise to behaviors that can threaten relationships and one's standing in the community:

#09: I've never had a good opinion of greedy people, people who only think about themselves. . . . I don't think that type of person is good for the community or for the family.

#01: One must learn to share, to work together, to have self-control. . . . I wouldn't want her to grow up with the "I deserve everything" mentality. There might be a time when she gets brushed off by others for such behavior.

#27: I wouldn't like them to be aggressive; on the contrary, I would like them to communicate and share. . . . Selfishness, to feel they are better than others, I don't like that either. I don't want them to be indifferent to others. If someone offers them their hand to shake, I want them to be thankful and *cariñosos*. . . . Just as people give them attention, they also should give people their attention without discrimination toward anyone. . . . I consider a person who [believes he is better than others] to be low. . . . You know, under my scale of values, he is not a complete human being.

The child who displays aggression, greed, and egotism thus runs the risk of rejection by the community for his or her lack of *respeto* and *cariño*. What must be controlled is therefore not so much an internal experience as its behavioral manifestation in relation to others. Emotions in and of themselves do not enhance or hinder the self; instead, it is the *expression* of emotions that must be monitored, lest they disrupt relationships. The desirability of being *tranquilo* also makes further sense in this context, inasmuch as it represents both attentive respectfulness and compliance, as well as self-control of the behavioral manifestations of inner negative emotions and desires:

> #12: But this one, I don't know how, she has the strongest will, she has the strongest will of all three [of my children]. With her everything is, "No, no, mama, no, father," and that is how she says it; she knows that she has a strong will. I would like for her to be *tranquila*, but that is just the way she is.

> #08: Well, I know a little girl, they have *educado* this one so badly, that she, well, she is a screamer, she does not behave herself, she cannot remain still next to her mother. . . . [She will not] remain *tranquila*. . . . She gets down off a chair, runs to pick up the toys, and the mother calls after her, "*Tranquilícese, tranquilícese, mira*" ("Calm down, calm down, look"), but she messes up all the toys.

In sum, whereas the Anglo mothers sought to help their children find an optimal balance between autonomy and relatedness, the Puerto Rican mothers hoped to instill in their children an understanding of the differing relational demands of *respeto*, *cariño*, and *confianza*. Inasmuch as a disobedient, restless child cannot exhibit Proper Demeanor, it was particularly important to the Puerto Rican mothers that their children be *obediente* and *tranquilo*. However, decorum is only one level of relatedness, and Puerto Rican mothers therefore also wanted their children to be able to bring a quality of positive emotional engagement (*cariño* and *confianza*) to their interactions when appropriate. This blend of Proper Demeanor and positive emotional engagement was viewed as prerequisite to someday becoming *una persona de provecho*—a person of worth, one who is trustworthy, compassionate, and useful to the community.

PERCEPTIONS OF ATTACHMENT BEHAVIOR

In our Study 2, both Anglo and Puerto Rican mothers were asked to give their impressions of six hypothetical toddlers in a simulated Strange Situation. Unlike the Anglo mothers, whose concern with a balance of autonomy and relatedness mapped easily onto the traditional conceptualization of Group A behavior as emotionally isolative, Group C behavior as lacking in autonomy, and Group B behavior as optimally balanced, the Puerto Rican mothers focused on the extent to which each toddler manifested Proper Demeanor. This consideration cut across traditional classification boundaries in unpredictable ways: Three of the toddlers, the A1, B1, and C1 toddlers, were considered to be lacking *respeto*.

Lack of *Respeto* and *Educacion*

Alex,[1] the active A1 toddler, was sharply criticized by the Puerto Rican mothers for his or her *intranquilo* behavior, a sign of poor manners and lack of *educacion* (proper upbringing). Such behavior reflects on the family:

> #312: She is one of these hyperactive children that can't stay *tranquila* or still anywhere. I wouldn't like my child to be like that, because then other people would say that I haven't *educado* my children. I think that this kid hasn't been *educado*.

> #319: Alex is a hyperactive and mischievous boy. I would not like my child to be like that, because they should learn how to behave in an office. If I do not *educar* them, then I would not feel fulfilled as a mother or as a child rearer.

> #324: She's too *intranquila*; she needs to be taught how to behave in an office. I wouldn't want my child to behave like this, because people would comment and say, "What a *vergüenza* that child is so *intranquila*." Imagine—if this is how she acts in an office, at home it must be even worse.

---

[1]Each of the hypothetical toddlers was given a Puerto Rican name, matched for the gender of each mother's Strange Situation-age child, in the Spanish versions of the vignettes. However, to eliminate confusion, we are using the gender-neutral English names only to describe mothers' perceptions of these toddlers.

#335: He's *malcriado*, naughty, meddlesome, touches everything; it all depends on how you *eduques* them and teach them; you have to teach them well; it's embarrassing when this happens; people say he's a little devil; you have to *educarlos* [bring them up properly].

The Puerto Rican mothers, then, were evaluating this A1 toddler along a dimension of behavior—activity level and the proper upbringing it indexes—not normally considered integral to the classification of attachment behavior; that is, an infant classified as A1 could be quiet as well as highly active. Similarly, a Group B or Group C infant could conceivably be just as active (or not) as this A1 infant. For instance, the active B1 toddler (Lee) was also disliked by the Puerto Rican mothers. Like Alex, Lee was considered to be *intranquilo* and lacking *educacion*—in short, a child who is overly active, noisy, disruptive to others, and a potential source of *vergüenza*:

#308: This behavior is like a hyperactive little girl's. I wouldn't like her to be like that, because if I go out anywhere with the little girl, then she would not behave appropriately. You have to teach children from the time they're very small.

#312: Lee is a mischievous boy, and hyperactive. I wouldn't like my child to be like that because then other people would say that I haven't *educado* them.

#327: She's too noisy with the toys; sometimes children do this to get attention from other people. I don't like this kind of behavior; people will say that you haven't taught them or *educado* them, and this will bring *vergüenza* to you.

#335: He's *intranquilo*, hyperactive, nervous, can't be quiet; [I wouldn't like it] because he brings you *vergüenza*, and this isn't good.

Finally, the C1 toddler, Lindsay, was also considered by the Puerto Rican mothers to be showing a lack of *respeto* and *educacion*. In Lindsay's case, however, this failure in Proper Demeanor manifested itself not so much in *intranquilo* behavior as in *malcriado* behavior. In particular, the Puerto Rican mothers viewed Lindsay's anger and willfulness as indicative of a child who lacks *respeto* and is therefore *malcriado*:

#313: *Malcriado*, because he probably misses his mother, but he shouldn't scream or throw anything to the floor. That is a poor attitude. [I wouldn't like it] because he shouldn't take the attitude of one who is *malcriado*. He can talk in a civilized manner, but not cry, scream, or throw.

#318: That Lindsay needs a spanking. He is *malcriado*. He is overly attached or spoiled. He is spoiled and *malcriado*. [I wouldn't like it] because he is a *malcriado* boy. He makes me feel *vergüenza* in front of people.

#323: *Malcriado*; doesn't want anything but the mother; [I wouldn't like it] because children should obey their parents, and if my child acted like this then I would be very *avergonzada* (ashamed).

#327: She's *malcriada*, pampered, and willful; [I wouldn't like it] because she wants to do whatever she wants. You have to teach them that they have to do what you say.

A lack of Proper Demeanor, then, dominated the reasons given by Puerto Rican mothers for finding the behavior of each of these three toddlers undesirable. Significantly, Proper Demeanor cuts across traditional attachment classification groups: The A1, B1, and C1 toddlers were all considered to lack proper *respeto* and *educacion*, the first two for their high activity level and the third for his or her willfulness and anger.

Does this, then, undercut the meaningfulness of Strange Situation behavior? One could speculate that virtually all Group C infants, who by definition show anger toward the primary caretaker, would be undesirable to the Puerto Rican mothers, suggesting that a Group C attachment pattern would be as maladaptive for Puerto Rican infants as it is for Anglo infants. On the other hand, the reasons *why* a Group C attachment pattern is maladaptive would appear to be culturally specific: For Anglo mothers it indexes a lack of autonomy and incapacity to cope with minor adversities, whereas for Puerto Rican mothers it manifests an inability to behave within culturally prescribed bounds of compliance and respect for authority. One could further hypothesize that a quiet Group A infant, although less undesirable than one who is *intranquilo*, would nonetheless cause concern because of his or her failure to acknowledge the mother's return (a lack of *respeto*) and nonengagement in the social environment (a lack of *cariño*). Indeed, this hypothesis receives partial confirmation from an earlier study of ours (Harwood & Miller, 1991), in which working-class migrant Puerto Rican mothers were critical of a quiet Group A infant's nonresponsiveness. Conversely, the child who is most desirable displays the requisite *respeto*, as well as an ability to engage in warm interpersonal relations.

Respeto and Cariño

The toddler who received the highest praise and desirability ratings from the island Puerto Rican mothers in Study 2 was Pat, the B3 toddler created on the basis of migrant Puerto Rican mothers' descriptions of desirable Strange Situation behavior. Pat was considered to display both *respeto* and *cariño*:

> #309: *Tranquila, educada, amable,* and *cariñosa;* she shows this when her mother comes back and she embraces her; my little girl is very *respetuosa* and *educada* like her, and she also is *cariñosa* with me.

> #319: Pat would be the ideal child for every mother. You can see that he is very *educado, amable,* and very attentive. Yes, [I would like this] because this child is very similar to my child. If you *educa* them and teach children how they should behave, then we will feel good.

> #324: She's *tranquila, obediente, respetuosa;* she seems *cariñosa,* a good girl; she's ideal for any mother; she's *tranquila* and *obediente.*

> #332: Very *tranquilo, educado,* he's been taught good manners; he loves his mother a lot and is *cariñoso.*

Thus, for both Puerto Rican and Anglo mothers, an optimal attachment pattern appeared most likely to be found within the Group B range of Strange Situation behavior. Yet, unlike our Anglo mothers, our Puerto Rican mothers conceptualized this optimal balance not in terms of autonomy and relatedness, but instead in terms of *respeto* and *cariño*—a contextually appropriate balancing of calm, respectful attentiveness with positive engagement in interpersonal relationships. Moreover, this balance does not represent a careful weighting of two fundamentally opposite tendencies (self vs. other), as it does in the Anglo mothers' perspective; instead, *respeto* and *cariño* are different levels of relatedness within the self's essential orientation toward others. What the child must learn is not how to maintain an inner balance of the polar ends of a teeter-totter, but rather what it is that particular social situations require in terms of *respeto, cariño,* and *confianza.* Thus, what is necessary is not an internal quality of "security" enabling the child to maintain this inner balance, but *educacion,* or upbringing in the contextually specific demands of proper demeanor. Moreover, whereas Group A and Group C Strange Situation behaviors were distinct for the Anglo mothers, representing opposite ends of a conceptual continuum, they were less so for the Puerto Rican mothers, for whom *respeto* could manifest itself in a variety of ways.

These findings are particularly noteworthy in light of Lamb et al.'s (1985) suggestion that although the major attachment classifications are treated as qualitatively different categories, they in fact may be conceptualized as falling along a continuum of behavior representing the relative balance between autonomy and relatedness: The two Group A patterns may represent high autonomy and low relatedness, the two Group C patterns may represent low autonomy and high relatedness, and the four Group B patterns may represent differing balances between the two. The present findings suggest that the balance between autonomy and relatedness is one useful way of conceptualizing the Strange Situation behavioral continuum—a way that also captures a central concern of socialization in Anglo-American culture. However, although the responses of the Puerto Rican mothers can be placed on this continuum, it is likely that the Puerto Rican mothers were attending primarily to dimensions of behavior (proper demeanor and positive engagement with the environment and other people) that are not captured in this conceptualization.

In fact, had the Strange Situation been conceived of originally by Puerto Rican rather than by Anglo psychologists, it is possible that highly active, angry, and externally distressed toddlers may have been grouped together at one end of the continuum as children who exhibit a lack of respectful attentiveness, whereas passively nonengaged, quietly avoidant, or extremely withdrawn toddlers may have been grouped together at the other end of the continuum as infants who fail to demonstrate joy or positive interest in others. In both conceptualizations, the desirable range of behavior would be in the Group B patterns. However, the continuum as a whole would be given culturally specific meaning that differentially defines its ends as well as its balanced middle. Moreover, the Puerto Rican mothers' concerns regarding activity level would make certain Group B toddlers (e.g., an active, distal B1 infant, such as Lee in this study) seem relatively undesirable, whereas the Anglo mothers' emphasis on self-maximization would render other Group B toddlers (e.g., a withdrawn, proximal B4 infant) similarly less desirable. Indeed, when middle-class Anglo and Puerto Rican mothers were asked in another study to rank-order specific preseparation Strange Situation behaviors, the Anglo mothers significantly preferred behaviors associated with active play, whereas the Puerto Rican mothers significantly preferred behaviors identified with sitting quietly (Harwood, Ventura-Cook, Schulze, & Wilson, 1995).

It must be emphasized here that there is a difference between the sense of safety provided by loving and attentive parents—a sense that may indeed universally predict the development of Group B versus non-B attachment patterns—and the psychological construct of inner security that is part and parcel of mainstream U.S. individualism. An infant may feel safe with his or her parents, and thus be "securely attached" in the classic sense of the term across all cultures; however, the construct of "security versus insecurity" has become equated in U.S. psychology with a host of culturally valued qualities that are specific to the socialization goals of our highly individualistic society, thus limiting their cross-cultural meaningfulness. Inasmuch as Group B Strange Situation behavior has been used as an indicator of culturally specific social competence as opposed to a potentially universal sense of safety, in that sense our interpretation of the meaningfulness of Strange Situation behavior is culturally bound.

When our Study 1 mothers were asked to describe what qualities they would like their children to possess as adults, 36% of middle-class and 60% of working-class Puerto Rican mothers' responses fell into the category of Proper Demeanor; this was the proportionally largest category of responses for both these groups, and significantly larger than any other single category. Similarly, when Study 1 mothers were asked what qualities they would *not* like their children to possess as adults, 48% of middle-class and 74% of working-class Puerto Rican mothers' responses fell once more into the category of Proper Demeanor—again, the proportionally largest category of responses for both these groups, and significantly larger than any other single category.

Proper Demeanor emerged again in Study 2 as the category most commonly used by both middle- and working-class Puerto Rican mothers when asked to evaluate the behavior of hypothetical toddlers in a simulated Strange Situation. For middle-class Puerto Rican mothers, four of the six toddlers (A1, B1, B3, and C1) elicited responses falling into the category of Proper Demeanor proportionally more than any other category (range = 35% to 64% of mothers' total number of responses). For working-class Puerto Rican mothers, five of the six toddlers (all but the B4) elicited responses falling into the category of Proper Demeanor proportionally more than any other category (range = 50% to 88% of mothers' total number of responses). In terms of desirability ratings, the Anglo mothers rated the active A1 and B1 toddlers as significantly more desirable than did the Puerto Rican mothers; conversely, as indicated above, Puerto Rican mothers rated the tranquil, affectionate B3 toddler as significantly more desirable than did the middle-class Anglo mothers.

The Place of Autonomy

Finally, it must be noted that considerations of autonomy were not absent among the Puerto Rican mothers, any more than concerns for filial cooperation and parental responsibility were entirely missing among the Anglo mothers. Indeed, among the Puerto Rican mothers, the category of Self-Maximization was proportionally larger than any other category in reference to the B4 infant, and proportionally similar to the Proper Demeanor category in reference to the B2 infant. On closer inspection, however, it is evident that the concern for autonomy expressed by the Puerto Rican mothers was not identical to the focus on Self-Maximization typical of the Anglo mothers. In particular, responses falling into the Self-Maximization category were, for the Puerto Rican mothers, more likely to center around a child's avoiding hardship by attaining some degree of independence than they were to emphasize the child's becoming a more completely realized individual:

> #01: I'm not going to live forever, and I have to let go of her. One day she will be on her own, and she has to take control of her life.

> #02: I would like them to . . . become independent; maybe the moment will come when they won't need me because I will be too old, and then I will be sure that they are going to be able to face their problems.

> #27: [I'd like them to possess] independence, because in the long run they are going to have to make it on their own. . . . There isn't always going to be someone there making decisions for them.

Similarly pragmatic concerns that a child develop some measure of autonomy emerged in the Puerto Rican mothers' perceptions of the clingy, distressed B4 toddler (Chris):

#308: Very attached to her mom; I wouldn't like my daughter to be so attached to me, because then if I had to go away and I had to leave her with somebody else, then she wouldn't be used to it and both of us would suffer.

#311: He's very dependent on his mother, close to her; I wouldn't like it because then we're both going to suffer if I need to leave him with another person, and he's unable to accept that.

#323: Pampered and attached to her mother. No, [I wouldn't like it] because I could never leave a child so attached to me; if I have to go some place that she can't, and I have to leave her with another person, then she's going to suffer a lot, and so will I.

#333: This child's pampered, attached to his mother, too attached to her, and this is bad for both of them; children suffer when they are so attached to their mothers, because if you have to leave them with other people, then they're going to cry a lot and they're going to suffer.

The Puerto Rican mothers, then, were not as concerned with autonomy as a component of a fully maximized individual; their concern stemmed from recognition that there are limits to a mother's ability to be continually present. A child who gains some measure of autonomy will suffer less when separations are necessary, and will be prepared to live without his or her parents' guidance following their eventual deaths. It would seem, therefore, that even when considerations of autonomy were present, they did not have the same cultural meaning for the Puerto Rican mothers that they did for the Anglo mothers.

Concepts of relatedness took on a similarly distinctive coloring. As the Anglo mothers saw it, relatedness is polar to and in tension with autonomy; a "secure" child is one who has the inner capacity to balance both these tendencies. In contrast, for the Puerto Rican mothers, relatedness was assumed; in their view, a child who is *educado* is not one who balances competing demands of self versus other, but one who knows which level of relatedness (*respeto, cariño, confianza*) is appropriate to which interpersonal setting, and how each dimension is best expressed in contextually specific ways.

CHAPTER SIX

Culture and Socioeconomic Status

◆

Many anthropologists have long recognized the importance of within-group variability, decrying the tendency to reify cultures and treat them as static, even homogeneous entities (Bourdieu, 1991; Roseberry, 1989; Sider, 1986). On the other hand, these same researchers have been equally quick to criticize those who would reduce all group variation to the functional requirements of social class. For instance, Geertz (1973) laments "the failure [of anthropology] to treat sociological and cultural processes on equal terms; almost inevitably one of the two is either ignored or is sacrificed to become but a simple reflex, a 'mirror image,' of the other. Either culture is regarded as wholly derivative from the forms of social organization . . . or the forms of social organization are regarded as behavioral embodiments of cultural patterns" (pp. 143–144).

The relationship between culture and social class is particularly problematic, given the nature of multiple and interpenetrating global influences in the world today. The romanticized, primitive Other, pure and untainted by the effects of modern civilization, survives now in the imagination rather than in reality. Some might argue that the increasingly pervasive effects of Westernization and industrialization have had or will have a homogenizing influence, thus reducing between-culture differences and creating instead a global system of working, middle, and upper classes, in which the classes at each level have more in common with one another than with their historical cultural traditions. If this is true, then it might seem that the more basic or "truer" unit of analysis is this global class system, rather than the historical cultural traditions within which the different socioeconomic groups around the world are embedded.

One of the problems with this issue has been the tendency to view cultures as isolable units or identifiable, internally coherent systems. If the term "culture" denotes an identifiable, internally coherent system, then how do we decide where to draw the boundaries that will tell us where one system ends and the next one begins? How much do two units need to have in common before we consider them part of the "same" culture, and, conversely, how much does one unit have to differ from another before it constitutes a separate entity? Is social class itself a cultural unit? If so, how does it relate to this larger entity we have called "dominant U.S. culture"?

DEVELOPMENTAL PSYCHOLOGY AND SOCIAL CLASS

Attention to social class differences within the field of anthropology has generally fallen to the anthropological subdiscipline called "political economy," which has traditionally used Marxist theory as a basis for tracing the historical processes assumed to be inherent in the separate, conflicting interests of the working and middle classes (see Roseberry, 1989; Wolf, 1982). Psychologists, however, have been more influenced by the sociological tradition of Max Weber, who articulated the idea that social stratification is best viewed as a graded series of status groups linked to one another in a relationship of inequality; these distinct but interrelated status groups share certain occupational, educational, and financial advantages or disadvantages (Jackman & Jackman, 1983; Powers, 1982). According to this view, the idea of "social class," which is based on the Marxist notion of the exploitation of one class by another, has to be distinguished from the concept of "socioeconomic status," which generally delineates a set of criteria in terms of which individuals may be ranked descriptively along a graded scale (Giddens, 1973). The measure constructed by Hollingshead (1975) is a good example of a scaling instrument that yields discrete socioeconomic status groups based on education and occupational prestige.

However, the terms "social class" and "socioeconomic status" have generally been and continue to be used interchangeably by psychologists to denote virtually any differences based on education, occupation, or income; this has given rise to considerable variability, if not confusion, within the literature regarding the definition and measurement of what we call "social class" (Hess, 1970; Hoff-Ginsberg & Tardif, 1995). Despite this variability, one consistent and robust finding with regard to child development has been that lower- or working-class parents (however defined) tend to place a relatively greater value than do middle-class parents (however defined) on obedience or conformity to authority, whereas middle-class parents tend to place a relatively greater value on initiative and self-direction (Gecas, 1979; Hoff-Ginsberg & Tardif, 1995; Kohn, 1977).

On the other hand, when Kohn (1977) extended his classic study of the relative valuing of initiative versus obedience among working- and middle-class parents to include Turin, Italy, he found that although class differences in Italy exist as they do in the United States, the cross-national differences obtained were greater than the within-culture class differences. Similarly, Perlmann (1988) examined ethnicity and class mobility in late 19th- and early 20th-century Providence, Rhode Island, and concluded that "cultural attributes and the [socioeconomic] situation in which [migrant ethnic groups] find themselves interact, [so] that it is foolish to think that either exists in a vacuum" (p. 8). In other words, the results of both these studies suggest that social class does not constitute a homogeneous global culture, any more than national culture does. As Roseberry (1988) notes, "anthropological subjects should be situated at the intersections of local and global histories. . . . [Researchers] must avoid making capitalism too determinative, and they must avoid romanticizing the cultural freedom of anthropological subjects" (pp. 173–174).

This idea is reiterated by several prominent social theorists who have argued that, however we finally define culture, it must be in such a way as to avoid the twin poles of reductionism—that is, conceiving of cultural differences purely in terms of economic and functional relations, or wholly in terms of reified meaning systems, without regard to the historical circumstances that have shaped ever-changing relationships among different socioeconomic groups (Blumer, 1990; Bourdieu, 1991; Giddens, 1973; Roseberry, 1988, 1989; Wolf, 1982). We arrive, then, at the question we began with: How are we to conceptualize the relationship between culture and the within-group variability we call "social class" or "socioeconomic status"? What exactly constitutes a cultural group?

CULTURE AS A CONTINUUM

One possibility, suggested by Cohen (1978), defines culture not as an isolable unit but as "a series of nesting dichotomizations of inclusiveness and exclusiveness. . . . [It is a process that is] both subjective and objective, [is] carried out by self and others, and depends on what diacritics are used to define membership. . . . The interactive situation is a major determinant of the level of inclusiveness employed in labeling self and others" (pp. 387–388). From this perspective, culture is a continuum involving levels of shared discourse. At the broadest, most inclusive level, we are all human beings who must confront the issues inherent in physical survival and attendant upon group or family life and the procreation of the species; we also all have relative access to an increasingly shared pool of information regarding globally marketed consumer products and international celebrities and events. We can all relate to one another on these levels. At the narrowest, most exclusive level, we are each absolutely unique individuals, and no two of us in the entire world are exactly alike.

In between these extremes are differing levels of shared discourse. Two U.S. residents, no matter how disparate their socioeconomic backgrounds, know generally how to conduct themselves around each other as polite strangers or as participants in a variety of culturally scripted activities, such as buying groceries, riding elevators, or ordering a meal at a restaurant. Moreover, no matter how disparate their backgrounds, most people living in the United States come to share a general belief in the importance of individual freedom and self-fulfillment, as well as the hope for upward mobility (Spence, 1985). Within those broad parameters, we each also maintain numerous other group memberships, entailing more narrow levels of shared discourse based on, among other things, geographic region, ethnicity, religion, political affiliation, gender, age, marital and parental status, sexual orientation, occupation, education, and avocation. Our personal identities are multiple and overlapping; we are simultaneously members of both a larger U.S. culture and a variety of smaller subcultures within that larger culture with which we identify. What changes as we move among these groups is not our cultural identities, but the markers we use to delineate the level of discourse appropriate to the situation we find ourselves in.

One major level of shared discourse is social class or socioeconomic status. In a national survey conducted by the Survey Research Center at the University of Michigan, using face-to-face interviews of

1,914 respondents from a random, multistage, probability-based sample of noninstitutionalized adults aged 18 and over residing in the 48 contiguous United States, Jackman and Jackman (1983) found not only that social class is a familiar concept to most U.S. residents, but also that substantial agreement exists concerning the association of different occupations with particular social classes. Moreover, based on their data, Jackman and Jackman suggest that "class has a subjective meaning that transcends the economic sphere and incorporates factors normally associated with status groups" (p. 41). In particular, two-thirds of the respondents considered beliefs, feelings, and style of life to be important criteria for membership in their own subjective social class. (In addition, subjective social class correlated quite strongly with objective social class as measured by occupational status.)

Social class thus appears to be a meaningful group membership to a majority of U.S. residents. If, however, members of different social classes or socioeconomic status groups also share in the larger U.S. culture, then one might reasonably ask whether broad cultural values of individual freedom, self-fulfillment, and upward mobility undergo specific, localized variations among different groups of people. Does the shared discourse of U.S. individualism take on more narrow meanings among specific groups? Similarly, does the shared discourse of Puerto Rican *respeto* take on more narrow meanings across different social classes in Puerto Rico? Concomitantly, if we find that working- and middle-class mothers generally differ in the relative value they place on conformity versus personal initiative, do these social class differences have culturally specific meanings in Connecticut as compared to Puerto Rico?

The hypothesis that U.S. individualism takes on specific, localized meanings among different socioeconomic groups finds support in the work of several psychologists who have studied working-class U.S. children and adults in recent years. Heath (1986) notes that working-class white and black parents believe as earnestly as do their middle-class counterparts that success in school will allow their children to "get ahead" in life, even while they provide them with markedly different experiences of extracting meaning from the written word. These differences translate into greater school success for middle-class children—an advantage that, though real, is not attributable to a greater belief in the value of schooling or "getting ahead," but to a different understanding of what patterns of behavior will lead to that end.

P. J. Miller (1982) similarly documents the way in which three working-class Baltimore mothers attempted to instill in their 2-year-old daughters skills of self-assertion and standing up for themselves, as well as learning how to control hurt feelings and getting their needs met. Although these goals were comparable to those expressed by the middle-class Anglo mothers in our study, the means—teasing, sometimes to the point of tears—was not. Strauss (1992) likewise describes how her working-class male interviewees "easily verbalized the values that underpin the 'American Dream': with hard work anyone in America can get ahead, and everyone should strive to do so" (p. 199). Yet the realities of day-to-day economic struggle rendered the security of a steady paycheck that would feed and house their families a more directive force in these men's lives than the lure of personal success and advancement. Finally, Schneider and Smith (1978), in their study of kinship, ideology, and social class in the United States, maintain that "middle-class values are dominant, both in the sense that middle-class patterns are upheld by the forces of the society as a whole . . . and in the sense that all classes pay symbolic deference to middle-class values while adhering to their own" (p. 3).

SOCIAL CLASS AND SELF-MAXIMIZATION AMONG ANGLO MOTHERS

In order to facilitate the interpretation of results in Study 1 regarding positive and negative adult and child characteristics, the four open-ended questions used were collapsed for further analysis. A 4×6 (group × category type) ANOVA yielded significant main effects for group, $F(3, 76) = 16.32, p < .01$, and category type, $F(5, 380) = 50.81$, $p < .01$, as well as a significant group × category type interaction, $F(15, 380) = 6.22, p < .01$.

A post hoc comparison of group means revealed that, compared to both Puerto Rican groups, both Anglo groups were more likely to use the Self-Maximization category, and middle-class Anglo mothers were less likely to use the Proper Demeanor category; in addition, working-class Anglo mothers were less likely than working-class Puerto Rican mothers to use the Proper Demeanor category. Moreover, a stepwise regression revealed that culture was the major predictor of group variance for three of the five categories: Self-Maximization, Self-Control, and Proper Demeanor (respective R^2 values = .48, .22, and .37).

The category of Self-Maximization includes the quality of self-direction or initiative, which Kohn (1977) argues is more highly valued by middle-class than by working-class parents. In our study, the category of Self-Maximization was indeed used at a significantly higher rate by the middle-class than by the working-class mothers (see Table 14). However, both middle- and working-class Anglo groups used this category significantly more than did either middle- or working-class Puerto Rican mothers (the four groups used this category across questions 45%, 32%, 17%, and 8% of the time, respectively).

As noted in previous chapters, the category of Self-Maximization broadly encompasses three dimensions of behavior, all of which are close to the heart of what is usually meant by a characterization of dominant U.S. culture as individualistic: independence, self-confidence, and personal achievement. As described in Chapter Four, these individualistic values were expressed at a relatively high rate by the Anglo mothers across social class. For instance, when asked to describe what qualities they would like their children to possess, many working-class mothers offered a list of potential skills to master and goals to accomplish:

> #164: Well, for one thing, neither me or his father graduated from high school. I would definitely like him to graduate from high school. And he already likes music, and I always wanted to play an instrument, and I would hope he plays the drums or the piano, because his father, too, always wanted to play the drums. So we hope that he will play the piano or anything he wants to play— any kind of musical instrument.

> #161: He's—he wants to go into gymnastics—he's doing it. He wants to be in baseball, he's doing—basketball, he's doing it.

TABLE 14. Mean Percentages of Category Usage across Questions, Study 1

Category	Anglo		Puerto Rican	
	Middle	Working	Middle	Working
Self-Maximization	45.3%	31.8%	17.4%	8.3%
Self-Control	18.0%	17.6%	11.4%	4.0%
Lovingness	14.4%	8.3%	16.2%	7.1%
Decency	5.0%	10.4%	12.7%	13.6%
Proper Demeanor	16.4%	31.2%	42.0%	66.9%
Miscellaneous	0.9%	0.7%	0.3%	0.1%

Note. Categories in Table 14 do not add up to 100% because of rounding.

He's only in kindergarten. And he's a straight A student. He's gonna be—he's 5½ and he has the mind of a 10-year-old. Proven by doctors and everything. So he's probably going to grow up being a genius, you know, which—good—you know, I don't mind that. But he's going for what he wants. He wants to be a gymnast.

#190: Umm, I'd like to see her have a good career when she grows up, and make lots of money (*laughs*), and, umm, I'd like to see her grow up to be a professional of some kind.

However, although Self-Maximization emerged as a major theme for the working- as well as the middle-class Anglo mothers, it was conceptualized by the working-class mothers from a somewhat different perspective. In particular, for many of the working-class mothers, the concern for Self-Maximization seemed to grow out of an acute awareness that this is what constitutes the "American dream"—a dream that they themselves had not achieved, but that they nonetheless hoped their children would. Often the vehicles for this were perceived to be education and a career:

#172: Well, I look at myself and I say I don't want her to be like that. I want her to further her career, you know, I want her to be able to read and write much better. Because, I mean, I guess I'm average, but I always wish I could have been further. But, uh, I guess that's what I want in her. I'd want her to further her career, like go to college, but reading and writing, really. I read to her a lot. I'd like her, you know, to know things a lot like that— her words and stuff.

#167: Well, they watch their father not working and stuff, so that's why my brother takes them [to work with him]: It shows them responsibility to work and stuff, which their father never did. . . . Like I'd rather them be independent and use their own— make their own decisions instead of following other people's decisions.

#173: Not to be like his father (*laughs*). No. Just to get ahead in life. [Could you say more?] Further his education, set goals for himself and be happy with them. . . . [You said you'd really not want him to be like his father.] (*laughs*) [What's his father like?] Well, his father—in with the wrong crowd, doing the wrong stuff, you know. I'm trying to bring him up in a better environment.

Put him away somewhere secluded (*laughs*). Bring him up in a better school, I guess—try and find him a better school.

For other working-class Anglo mothers, the concern that their children develop their inner potential seemed rooted in a perception of the realities of life in the United States:

#175: Oh, I'm really concerned about teaching her things. We watch *Sesame Street* every day. Because they have to be really prepared for kindergarten and stuff. So she can say A, B, C, and count 1, 2, 3, 4, 5.

#162: If it was, you know, for me to decide if—I'd like him to go to college and be something, you know. I'd really like him to make something out of his life, you know, something that is going to have a little money in it, because that's exactly what you need these days.

#174: I'd definitely like her to be independent. Umm, happy-go-lucky. Looking for a good education. Not relying on the fact that "I'm gonna grow up and I'm gonna get married and raise a family." Sort of the roles—it's different now.

Thus, across socioeconomic status, the Anglo mothers in this study expressed substantial concern that their children develop the skills and abilities to "get ahead in life." However, this concern took on a specific, localized meaning among the working-class Anglo mothers, which seemed to reflect an acute awareness of the difficulty they themselves had encountered in trying to realize the "American dream" of success, as well as a desire that their children might succeed where they had not. Perhaps this awareness is related to the lesser usage of the Self-Maximization category by the working-class than by the middle-class Anglo mothers: When a particular goal—even one as societally prescribed as the "American dream"—becomes less obtainable, then often other, more realizable goals and values gain greater salience. Alternatively, one could speculate that these mothers grew up placing more emphasis on other goals (either by personal predilection or by family example), and that they were thus recreating as adults an environment in which other goals and values both had greater cognitive prominence and were expressed in their life choices. At any rate, whatever the direction of causality, the working-class Anglo mothers in our study endorsed the mainstream U.S. success model for their children, even while they both verbalized and lived out other, less success-oriented goals and values.

SOCIAL CLASS, PROPER DEMEANOR, AND DECENCY AMONG ANGLO MOTHERS

The two categories used more often by working-class than by middle-class Anglo mothers to describe qualities they would like their children to possess were Proper Demeanor and Decency. The category of Proper Demeanor subsumes the quality of obedience, or conformity to authority, which Kohn (1977) concludes is more highly valued by working-class than by middle-class parents. Indeed, consistent with Kohn's findings, the working-class Anglo mothers in this study evidenced a higher usage of the Proper Demeanor category across questions (31%) than did the middle-class Anglo mothers (16%), although both Anglo groups used this category across questions less often than did the two Puerto Rican groups (67% and 42% for working- and middle-class Puerto Rican mothers, respectively).

The use of the Proper Demeanor category among working-class Anglo mothers depended, however, in large part on whether they were referring to long-term goals or to child behavior. In particular, a concern for Proper Demeanor among these mothers surfaced only about 20% of the time in response to the questions concerning long-term goals, but accounted for roughly 40% of their total responses when describing desirable and undesirable *child* behavior:

> #169: She's excellent. When I babysit for her, and she comes here, it's like she'll watch the baby, she'll be cleaning the house—she'll do everything for me. She is so good. You don't even mind having her at all. She's quiet and she'll do anything to help you out.

> #191: When she's over at your house, you don't have to worry that she'll be fresh or wreck anything. She plays nice and she's always "please" and "thank you"; she's polite with her manners. That's what I like.

> #161: Yeah, I know this little kid that I wouldn't want my kid hanging around with him. . . . He doesn't listen. He'll swear up a storm. He's 4 years old, and he's swearing, he's like—he's wearing leathers already, acting like he's big and bad. I don't like that. That's not me. [So it's like he's—] He's rebellious.

The working-class Anglo mothers used the Proper Demeanor category twice as often when describing child behavior as they did when describing long-term socialization goals. The examples given above were typical, in that they tended to involve behaviors that made an adult's life more or less pleasant. Children might be "good," quiet, easy to handle, and helpful, or they might be obstreperous, defiant, and obnoxious. This may have reflected a concern for conformity to authority that was functionally related to working-class occupational status, as hypothesized by Kohn. However, it may also have reflected either (1) concern for the presence of childhood precursors (such as "swearing up a storm" and "wearing leathers") of being sidetracked into drugs and crime as adolescents and young adults, a concern reflected in their relatively greater use of the Decency category; or (2) high stress levels in the lives of the working-class mothers in this sample, many of whom were single parents, and all of whom were financially strained. These mothers may have wanted their children to develop their individual potential, but they may also have had a greater need than the middle-class Anglo mothers had for their children to engage in behavior that would contribute to household calm and orderliness.

As in the case of the Proper Demeanor category, working-class Anglo mothers were more likely than middle-class Anglo mothers to use the category of Decency; the dimension of behavior captured by this category is that of an upstanding citizen who lives an honest, hardworking life and abides by the laws of society. However, working-class Anglo mothers' greater use of the Decency category—unlike that of the Proper Demeanor category—emerged only in reference to long-term goals, particularly *undesirable* long-term goals. In fact, working-class Anglo mothers used the Decency category 25% of the time when describing undesirable long-term goals (see Table 3):

#161: I don't want them like turning out like druggies, or hanging around with people that are no good.

#171: Drug addicts. Just all the bad things I don't want them to be. [What would some of those be?] Hanging around with the wrong kind of people, getting into trouble, stuff like that.

#190: I had friends that got to be like in the seventh, eighth grade, they thought it was cool to shoplift. I don't want her to try any of that stuff. Uh, she's been getting how bad drugs are dumped into her head since she was about 3 weeks old (*laughs*), umm, things like that. Because I grew up in a very nice neighborhood, but most of the kids I went to grammar school with, all the boys are in jail now; the girls have been there too.

#192: I'd have to worry about the clientele he hangs around with, the people he brings home, the families they come from, what he learns on the school bus. Drugs, weapons—it's scary, but you have to confront it as you see it.

Middle-class Anglo mothers showed little tendency to use the Decency category at all; in fact, it accounted across questions for only about 5% of their total responses. On the other hand, it seems likely that, if asked, middle-class Anglo mothers would also have expressed a desire for their children not to end up on drugs or in prison. It is possible to spectulate that this heightened concern among the working-class Anglo mothers that their children avoid "all the bad things" may have reflected in part the realities of their lives. The working-class mothers were substantially poorer and more likely to be living in neighborhoods with a high crime rate, as well as high school dropout and unemployment rates. It is conceivable that drug dealing emerges much more openly in such neighborhoods as an economic alternative to conventional employment. The answers that the working-class Anglo mothers gave may thus have reflected the greater salience of drugs and crime in their lives—a salience echoed also, as described above, in the extent to which the goals of Self-Maximization were viewed as in part pragmatically necessary (a person needs money and "smarts" to survive in life), but also as potentially problematic (they hoped their children would "do better" than they had done, but there are no guarantees in life).

SOCIAL CLASS AND PROPER DEMEANOR AMONG PUERTO RICAN MOTHERS

As described above, the Proper Demeanor category subsumes the qualities of obedience and conformity to authority, which Kohn (1977) found to be more highly valued by working-class than by middle-class parents. Consistent with Kohn's (1977) findings, working-class Puerto Rican mothers used the Proper Demeanor category more than did middle-class Puerto Rican mothers, accounting respectively for 67% and 42% of their total number of responses across the four open-ended questions. However, both groups of Puerto Rican mothers used this category across questions more than did either Anglo group. Moreover, unlike the Anglo mothers, the Puerto Rican mothers were as likely to use the Proper Demeanor category when describing long-term adult socialization goals as they were when characterizing child behavior. In other words, proper demeanor was held to be an essential quality of the well-socialized adult, and not just of the well-behaved child; as such, it went beyond the simple dimension of obedience or conformity to authority. As discussed in Chapter Five, both middle- and working-class Puerto Rican mothers viewed their children as living their lives under the watchful eyes of an observing community, which has the power to offer either love and acceptance or rejection and pain:

> #57: [I want her to be] *respetuosa* because like I was saying, I want others to *respetar* her also . . . because if [my children] were *malcriados* or sexually loose, then people wouldn't accept them, nor would others *respetar* them or accept them, or look well on them; they would be rejected.

> #10: [I would not like my children] to be *malcriados* . . . [because then] people wouldn't love them. They would be despised. No one would love them. They would earn the hatred of others. . . . No one would do them any favors; no one would trust them.

This concern among the Puerto Rican mothers in our study cut across social class. However, it is interesting to note that whereas among Anglo mothers the category containing culturally valued qualities associated with individualism was expressed at the highest rate among middle-class mothers, among Puerto Rican mothers the category containing culturally valued qualities associated with a more sociocentric orientation was expressed at the highest rate among working-class mothers. It should also be noted that middle-class Anglo and Puerto Rican mothers used these major cultural categories at almost identical rates: Across questions, 45% of the middle-class Anglo mothers' responses fell into the Self-Maximization category, while 42% of the middle-class Puerto Rican mothers' responses fell into the Proper Demeanor category. What differed was the direction of the working-class mothers' "deviation" from the middle-class "norms": Working-class Anglo mothers expressed a smaller percentage of Self-Maximization responses, whereas working-class Puerto Rican mothers expressed a greater percentage of Proper Demeanor responses.

We have speculated earlier that the harsher socioeconomic realities of working-class Anglo mothers' lives have made the attainment of culturally valued individual success more problematic; moreover, as individual success became more illusory, other goals (such as good behavior in childhood and personal decency in adulthood) may have gained greater salience in comparison. However, there is no comparable trend or argument to make among the Puerto Rican mothers. The category of Proper Demeanor, which contains culturally valued qualities associated with a sociocentric orientation, was used more rather than less by the working-class compared to the middle-class Puerto Rican mothers. In addition, Proper Demeanor would not seem to be either easier or more difficult to achieve by one group or the other. For instance, none of the Puerto Rican mothers spoke wistfully of how they wished they had had more of an opportunity to learn *respeto* when they were young, or hoped that their children would have more of it than they did. Similarly, neither class group expressed a greater or lesser awareness than the other group that *respeto* is needed to survive in their world: Puerto Rican mothers across social class seemed acutely aware of this, and the importance and difficulties of instilling it in children were expressed by both groups.

What did seem to distinguish the middle- from the working-class Puerto Rican mothers was the working-class mothers' nearly exclusive, single-minded focus on the category of Proper Demeanor. Across questions, fully two-thirds of the working-class Puerto Rican mothers' responses fell into the Proper Demeanor category; the second greatest percentage of category usage was Decency, at 14%, with the usage of the remaining categories all falling under 10%. In contrast, the middle-class Puerto Rican mothers used the Proper Demeanor category just under half the time, with the rest of their responses spread fairly evenly among the remaining categories. In particular, working-class Puerto Rican mothers were across questions less likely than the middle-class Puerto Rican mothers to use the Self-Control (4% and 11% of total responses, respectively), Lovingness (7% and 16% of total responses, respectively), and Self-Maximization (8% and 17% of total responses, respectively) categories.

SOCIAL CLASS AND SELF-MAXIMIZATION AMONG PUERTO RICAN MOTHERS

Consistent with Kohn's (1977) findings, middle-class Puerto Rican mothers used the Self-Maximization category more than did working-class Puerto Rican mothers (see the percentages just above). However, also as noted above, both groups of Puerto Rican mothers used this category less than did either Anglo group. This tendency among the middle-class Puerto Rican mothers emerged most strongly in descriptions of positive behavior, both long-term adult goals as well as positive child behavior, where it accounted for nearly 25% of their total responses. However, whereas the Anglo mothers used the category of Self-Maximization to express a desire that their children realize their full potential as self-confident, autonomous, and creative individuals, the use of this category by middle-class Puerto Rican mothers reflected a concern that their children grow into responsible adults able to make important life decisions:

> #01: I can guide her while she is young, make decisions for her, decide for her, but she must—the day will arrive when she will have to make decisions. In fact, she does make decisions, not very important ones—she decides what she wants to eat, what she wears—but eventually she must become responsible, determine her own future, and accept the consequences of the decisions that she makes. Her being responsible for her life is very important.

> #02: [I'd like] that at the moment they make a decision in any critical situation that has to do with their future, then I hope they will know how to decide what is best. This is what I'd like: enough wisdom to let them be sure of the next step they are taking—that they not be indecisive when they have to make a serious decision, and that it be the correct one.

> #27: Now they are children, but afterwards when they are adults, [independence] is something that will allow them to choose the path of good by themselves. They will know how to differentiate between the good and bad, because there isn't always going to be someone there making decisions for them.

For the middle-class Puerto Rican mothers, then, the development of independence was important, but was associated more with the demands of becoming a responsible adult than with the pursuit of one's full individual potential. Doing well in school as a child was similarly linked for these mothers with the development of responsibility, as opposed to the advancement of individual success:

> #06: This girl has all the characteristics of a responsible child— she worries a lot about her homework; since she was a little girl she's taken responsibility.

#33: There are some children in the school who are very irresponsible. They do not have good study habits. Their physical appearance is always very dirty. They do not write anything. They don't do assignments, are very poorly brought up. I do not know what their problem is, but they are very behind, far behind everyone.

#57: Responsible, very responsible, especially about school matters, homework. She comes home and quickly does her homework. She tells me, "Mom, I have homework." She worries a lot about being responsible, especially academically. She is affectionate and adorable.

Other qualities included within the category of Self-Maximization (e.g., security, intelligence, achieving goals) were depicted by the middle-class Puerto Rican mothers either as in potential conflict with one's life in the community, or as a way to serve others better:

#01: You can't just order people to think and act as you do. You lay out your goals, you want to achieve things. You go to a job and you want to fix a whole lot of things that are wrong. But you cannot just assume that since you have a clear perception of things or because you have knowledge about something because you just graduated, then things have to be done in a certain way just as you wish. What happens then, if things aren't done as you wish? You become impatient and you could even be disrespectful to a colleague.

#06: Intelligence [is] a beautiful quality that he should have in order to get along with others.

#30: [What other qualities would you like them to have as they are growing up?] That they keep being interested in school. [Why?] So that they will study—so they will study and have a good future, so they have a future—a good job, so they can support their mother.

#37: I would like [him] to be intelligent, good, and obedient. That way he would be developing; for me, he would know how to relate to people.

In short, the use of the Self-Maximization category by the middle-class Puerto Rican mothers was not identical to that of the middle-class Anglo mothers, but instead reflected more culturally specific concerns. Although middle-class Puerto Rican mothers used the Self-Maximization category more than did working-class Puerto Rican mothers, this did not translate into an endorsement of the Self-Maximization construct as described by Anglo middle-class mothers. Independence was viewed as a part of responsibility; intelligence was seen as important for knowing how to get along with others; getting a good job would secure not only children's own future but that of their aging parents. Similar trends occurred with the middle-class Puerto Rican mothers' use of the Self-Control and Lovingness categories:

#02: [I wouldn't like them to be] vain, that they believed themselves to be—that they deserve such a thing, that they cannot live without certain things, without certain luxuries. I would not like them to grow up in that environment, or believing that they are better than other people; what I mean is that we are all at the same level. That they learn not to be impatient. That everything has its time, its place, that everything will come true, all the things that they hope for. But above all, I would not like them to think that they are better than anybody else, or that material things take priority.

#11: [I wouldn't like him to] believe he is better than others, that he be proud in the sense that he doesn't want to share with the other children and he doesn't want to socialize with them because he sees them as inferior to him. I wouldn't like him to think he didn't have to share with other children because they belonged to a different social class. You know, because he is poorer or because this one is black or this other one is not black. I truly would not support that; I would definitely not support that. I wouldn't support him being proud like that toward anyone in the world, and that he didn't have the grace, you know, to greet people.

#27: I wouldn't like them to be aggressive; on the contrary, I would like them to communicate and share. I wouldn't like them to be selfish; again, I would like them to share, that they don't go around differentiating the good things that they have versus the bad things someone else has, also the bad things they have versus the good things others have. I don't like those comparisons. Selfishness, to feel they are better than others, I don't like that either. I don't want them to be indifferent to others. If someone offers them their hand to shake, I want them to be thankful and *cariñosos*.

In other words, when middle-class Puerto Rican mothers used the Self-Control and Lovingness categories, their concerns were not identical to those voiced by the Anglo mothers. As described in Chapter

Four, Anglo mothers tended to view Lovingness and Self-Control in relation to Self-Maximization: Do the relevant qualities enhance or hinder its realization? In contrast, the middle-class Puerto Rican mothers tended to view Self-Control and Lovingness in relation to Proper Demeanor: Does a child treat others with forbearance, respect, and generosity, and thus gain esteem and affection in the community?

Analogously, although working-class Anglo mothers used the Proper Demeanor category more than did middle-class Anglo mothers, they generally used only selected aspects of it (e.g., a child who does what he or she is told, doesn't talk back, and helps out around the house), and not the fully elaborated construct as it exists in Puerto Rico: living under the watchful eyes of the observing community, acting with *respeto* in order to gain esteem and avoid *vergüenza*, and being *una persona de provecho*.

SOCIAL CLASS AND CULTURE

In conclusion, although class variability existed in our samples in the direction hypothesized by Kohn (1977), the cultural categories of Self-Maximization and Proper Demeanor encompassed far more than simply "initiative versus conformity to authority," and class differences appeared to take shape in culturally specific directions.

Working-class Anglo mothers had experienced the difficulty of attaining the upwardly mobile success characteristic of the "American dream," and appeared concomitantly to give other qualities more weight. Their greater emphasis on good behavior in childhood and decency in adulthood may have reflected salient socioeconomic factors in their lives, and may also have been an attempt to define for themselves a different standard of personal worth. As Strauss (1992) notes of her U.S. working-class male interviewees, "Although my interviewees voiced [the American] success model, they appear to hold it in a bounded way" (p. 199). Similarly, the working-class Anglo mothers endorsed the qualities falling within the category of Self-Maximization, but these qualities also seemed somewhat at variance with the realities of their own lives; they dealt with this discrepancy both by expressing the hope that their own children would be able to eliminate it, and by adhering at the same time to a somewhat different set of standards by which to measure personal worth.

Unlike their Anglo counterparts, working-class Puerto Rican mothers appeared to experience no dissonance between the culturally valued qualities associated with a more sociocentric perspective, and what motivated their daily lives. In fact, they used the category of Proper Demeanor at a far higher rate than did the middle-class Puerto Rican mothers. What distinguished the two Puerto Rican groups was not that the working-class mothers had to reconcile major cultural values with the socioeconomic realities of their lives, but that the middle-class mothers made greater use of other categories focusing more on the individual and his or her internal life (i.e., Self-Maximization, Self-Control, and Lovingness). This may have reflected the reality of being in jobs that require more self-direction, as proposed by Kohn; or it may have reflected either a higher degree of "Americanization" among the educated Puerto Rican mothers, or a Maslowian freedom to examine the inner person to a greater degree once the basic needs of survival are met. In addition, it is important to note that the middle-class Puerto Rican mothers' greater use of the categories of Self-Maximization, Self-Control, and Lovingness seemed to occur in culturally prescribed ways, and not simply as Puerto Rican counterparts of the middle-class Anglo ideal.

One could also argue that the mothers sorted themselves into different social strata on the basis of their individual predilections, and that once they were immersed in the lifestyle associated with a given social strata, their beliefs would find confirmation among others choosing a similar lifestyle (Scarr, 1992). However, the point here is not to establish direction of causality, but to note the following:

1. Socioeconomic status appeared to be associated with the relative valuing of Proper Demeanor and Self-Maximization among both the Anglo and the Puerto Rican mothers.

2. The culturally valued constructs of Proper Demeanor and Self-Maximization represented far more than a simple dichotomy between personal initiative and conformity to authority, thus giving rise to cross-cultural differences in the use of these two categories that were at least as large as the within-group differences.

3. The within-group variability that we call "social class" produced different tensions in relation to major cultural constructs among Anglo as compared to Puerto Rican mothers. In particular, whereas working-class Anglo mothers appeared more ambivalent than did middle-class Anglo mothers in their endorsement of the mainstream U.S. success model, the working-class Puerto Rican mothers seemed more single-mindedly focused than did middle-class Puerto Rican mothers on the importance of Proper Demeanor.

4. Mothers' use of all the categories, as well as the socioeconomic

differences themselves, appeared to be embedded within their respective cultural traditions.

In this sense, as Roseberry (1988) observes, these middle- and working-class Anglo and Puerto Rican mothers were all "situated at the intersections of local and global histories" (p. 173). They were each immersed within historical cultural traditions that shaped many of their beliefs regarding long-term socialization goals and child behavior, even while those beliefs were undergoing specific modifications in relation to different socioeconomic concerns. Working-class Anglo mothers held ideals of personal success in tension with other salient goals and self-definitions, while middle-class Anglo mothers appeared to be spokeswomen of the virtues and potential within the "American dream." Working-class Puerto Rican mothers championed the Puerto Rican value of *respeto*, while middle-class Puerto Rican mothers sought to integrate alternative conceptualizations into the complex web of traditional values. Neither socioeconomics nor a national reified meaning system proved to be wholly determinative or homogenizing.

One could further note that within each socioeconomic "group" were additional divisions, based on, among other things, geographic region, ethnicity, religion, political affiliation, gender, age, marital and parental status, sexual orientation, occupation, education, and avocation. The use of distinct groups for analytic or comparative purposes lends substance to the myth that cultures exist as isolable units with identifiable boundary markers that tell us where one "culture" ends and the next begins. However, if culture is a continuum, then the boundary markers we erect for analytic or comparative purposes are arbitrary and depend on the level of analysis we wish to engage in, and not on any naturally occurring series of fundamental units. From this, we conclude that there is a broad level at which we can speak of "Anglo" versus "Puerto Rican" culture, just as there is another, narrower level at which we can describe "working-class Anglo" compared to "middle-class Anglo" culture. Within each of these are further group divisions that would allow us to do increasingly fine-grained analyses, based on differing levels of shared history, experience, and discourse.

SOCIAL CLASS, CULTURE, AND PERCEPTIONS OF ATTACHMENT BEHAVIOR

Mothers' perceptions of the six hypothetical toddlers in the simulated Strange Situation in Study 2 showed the same patterns of within-group variability as did their open-ended descriptions of socialization goals. In particular, middle-class mothers were more likely than working-class mothers to use the Self-Maximization category to describe what they did or didn't like about the toddlers, whereas working-class mothers were more likely than middle-class mothers to use the Proper Demeanor category. On the other hand, this within-group variability occurred within a context of cross-cultural differences in which Puerto Rican mothers in general were more likely to use the Proper Demeanor category than were Anglo mothers, who in turn were more likely to use the Self-Maximization category. In fact, cross-cultural differences in the percentages of category usage were even more pronounced in mothers' perceptions of attachment behavior than they had been in their descriptions of socialization goals and child behavior (see Table 14).

In addition to general differential usage of the Self-Maximization and Proper Demeanor categories, differences in the use of the Self-Control and Lovingness categories arose in specific instances. In particular, Anglo mothers were more likely than Puerto Rican mothers to use the Self-Control category when describing the C1 toddler. In this instance, Anglo mothers showed almost identical usage of the Self-Control category (38%); in contrast, a class difference emerged among Puerto Rican mothers, with middle- and working-class Puerto Rican mothers using this category in 26% and 17% of their responses, respectively.

The findings regarding the use of the Lovingness category are similarly complex and contextual. For two of the toddlers (A1 and B1), both class and culture effects emerged, with Anglo mothers and middle-class mothers more likely to use this category than Puerto Rican mothers and working-class mothers. For the other toddlers, however, class effects appeared in one culture but not another, or cultural differences appeared in one social class but not the other. In general, however, middle-class Anglo mothers used the Lovingness category more, and working-class Puerto Rican mothers used this category less, than did any of the other groups. These findings suggest that whereas the culture and class differences in the use of the Self-Maximization and Proper Demeanor categories appeared to be relatively robust, group differences in the use of other categories may have been more contextually bound and related in complex ways to both culture and class considerations.

CHAPTER SEVEN

Attachment, Culture, and Behavior

♦

In the last several chapters, we have examined Anglo and Puerto Rican mothers' perceptions of desirable and undesirable attachment behavior; in so doing, we have used a symbolic approach, which seeks to relate perceptions of relative desirability to mothers' long-term socialization goals and cultural meaning systems. In the past, cross-cultural attachment research has generally taken an adaptationist approach, and attempted to relate different patterns of attachment to the adaptive behavioral demands of a specific ecological niche. However, as several researchers have noted, important to all human ecological niches are the symbolic meaning systems that serve to transmit much of what we call "culture"; much of this transmission process is accomplished through everyday interactional routines between caretakers and children (Harkness et al., 1992; Schieffelin & Ochs, 1986; Tomasello et al., 1993). Just as children abstract the rules of their native language from relevant contexts and then begin to use those rules to generate novel sentences, so children abstract from everyday interactions the social norms of their cultural group, and then reconstruct those norms in their own interactions. Similarly, just as the generation of novel sentences by competent speakers can introduce change into a language, so can the reconstruction of social norms by competent actors lead to alterations in those norms. Continuity and change are thus both entailed in this model. According to this view, the language and nonverbal communications used by caretakers to organize interactions are key to understanding the processes by which children become socially competent members of a given cultural group.

Concomitantly, as D'Andrade and Strauss (1992) and Harkness and Super (1992) suggest, these meaning systems or "parental ethnotheories" also have motivational properties, and so function as goals as well as interpretations of reality.

Although the studies presented in this book have not examined cultural differences in the interactional routines that serve to organize the attachment system, they have sought to explore the influence of cultural meaning systems on mothers' perceptions of the relative desirability of different patterns of attachment behavior. In terms of adult perceptions and interpretations, Levy (1980) and Malatesta and Haviland (1985) have suggested that cultural groups vary in the extent to which certain emotional experiences and behaviors are either conceptually elaborated on (hypercognized as positive goals to be sought after or as negative experiences to be avoided) or conceptually minimized as relatively unimportant (hypocognized). These conceptual frameworks make certain emotional experiences more or less available to reflective consciousness for members of different cultural groups, depending on whether they are hypercognized or hypocognized. In this way, cultural meaning systems provide the conceptual frameworks that are likely to be used to interpret emotional cues and experiences. For instance, for Anglo-Americans "self-esteem" and "insecurity" appear to comprise hypercognized constructs, whereas for Puerto Ricans the experiences of *respeto* ("respect") and *vergüenza* ("shame") are hypercognized (Crespo, 1986; Harwood, 1992; Lauria, 1982). Thus, objectively similar situations will be interpreted and evaluated differently, depending on whether one's conceptual and phenomenological focus is on personal inadequacy or on public loss of face.

In addition, culturally different conceptual structures for the understanding of different behaviors and emotions not only shape the interpretation and evaluation of one's own experience (Lewis, 1989); they also serve as a framework for interpreting the actions of others. In other words, one not only interprets one's own experiences in relation to the hypercognized constructs of a given sociocultural group, but also interprets the actions of others according to these constructs. Social interactions themselves are thus mediated by the cultural constructs we use to understand both self and other. For instance, it will matter a great deal to the interpretation and negotiation of everyday social interactions whether a toddler's active play is interpreted positively by caretakers as exploration and curiosity, according to a cultural construct that places the greatest value on Self-Maximization; or whether it is interpreted negatively as being *intranquilo* (restless), according to a cultural construct that places the greatest value on Proper Demeanor and dignity in social relations.

Finally, as several researchers have suggested (D'Andrade & Strauss, 1992; Sigel, McGillicuddy-DeLisi, & Goodnow, 1992), inasmuch as these meaning systems "not only label and describe the world but also set forth goals (both conscious and unconscious) and elicit or include desires" (Strauss, 1992, p. 3), they provide a motivational link between interpretations or perceptions and actual parental behavior. For instance, in their examination of parental ethnotheories and the developmental niche among U.S. mothers in Cambridge, Massachusetts, and Kipsigis mothers in Kokwet, Kenya, Harkness and Super (1992) found that the Cambridge children between the ages of 1 and 5 years spent over half their waking time engaged in activities involving play, TV/books, and bedtime rituals with their parents, but less than 1% of their time doing household chores. In contrast, the Kokwet children aged 3 to 6 years spent nearly a quarter of their time doing chores. Harkness and Super relate these differences in the everyday activities of Cambridge and Kokwet children to the differences in cultural values and goals expressed by the parents. In particular, the Cambridge mothers placed a great deal of emphasis on the development of cognitive capacities and self-reliance. They believed that playing would contribute to the development of imagination, creativity, and other cognitive skills, and encouraged their children to spend time in these activities. In addition, time spent alone in play was thought to enhance or demonstrate independence. On the other hand, the Kokwet mothers showed more concern for the development of responsibility and obedience, and the greater time spent by Kokwet children on household chores reflects this developmental goal. Harkness and Super conclude that parental meaning systems not only provide a framework for interpreting the child's behavior, but also give motivational force to the organization of everyday activities and the encouragement of some behaviors over others.

With regard to emotions, several researchers have noted that the capacity for and potential range of expressive behavior in the human neonate are biologically determined (Dixon, Tronick, Keefer, & Brazelton, 1981; Harkness & Super, 1985; Lewis & Saarni, 1985). Similarly, states of arousal in infancy, such as distress or relaxation, are not cultural creations. However, these same researchers have suggested that this universal repertoire of arousal states and behaviors is culturally shaped (see Malatesta & Haviland, 1985; Lewis, 1989). In particular, the display rules regarding the expression of different emotions vary across different groups; that is, culturally diverse norms exist regarding the extent to which certain emotions are either heightened or dampened in their display. For instance, J. L. Briggs (1970) describes the extent to which the Inuit value mildness in affective displays, and the concomitant subtlety with which they express anger—a subtlety that Briggs reports led her initially to underestimate the impact of seemingly mild reprimands on young Inuit children. Dixon et al. (1981) similarly describe cultural regulations regarding the expression of intense emotions among the Gusii. It thus appears that parents' expressive interactions with their infants reflect from birth these larger cultural norms and patterns regarding the context for and interpretation of appropriate emotional display.

There are at least two implications of this research for the cultural study of attachment. First, parent–infant interactions occur from birth within a matrix of meanings that serves to shape a universal human capacity for social, emotional, and linguistic expressiveness into culturally specific elaborations, attenuations, and conceptualizations. In this way, even before the second-year speech explosion, infants have begun to learn to produce and respond to the basic interpersonal norms that will organize and inform their social interactions throughout their lives. From this perspective, a culturally sensitive approach to Strange Situation behavior needs to proceed on the basis of indigenous understandings of the interactional norms and socioemotional display rules that begin to shape the expressive behavior of children from birth, and that affect the interpretation and consequent management of those behaviors by adult caretakers.

Second, these culturally specific interactional norms and socioemotional display rules are part of a larger web of cultural meanings regarding conceptions of the self and other. As Lutz and White (1986, p. 417) observe, "concepts of emotion emerge as a kind of language of the self—a code for statements about intentions, actions, and social relations." Moreover, the task of interpreting a central cultural emotion term (e.g., the Ilongot term *liget* or "anger," the Puerto Rican term *respeto* or "respect," and the American term "self-esteem") can be "virtually indistinguishable from the ethnography itself, requiring a mapping of multiple usages across a variety of social contexts" (p. 423), and thus intertwining understanding of the experience of the self with an understanding of the behavior of others. From this standpoint, perceptions of Strange Situation behavior afford a window into cultural meanings regarding interactional norms and their interpretation. In this way, some of the central constructs of a given sociocultural group—its frameworks for interpreting and evaluating socio-emotional behavior—can be elucidated.

It is important to note in this regard that Bowlby hypothesized that the child's cognitions (or the internal working models built up on the basis of repeated interactions with primary caretakers) play an important mediating role in individual differences in attachment behavior (Bowlby, 1980; Bretherton, 1985). However, the parent–infant interactional routines that contribute to the formation of internal working models are themselves influenced not only by idiographic life experiences, but by larger cultural constraints as well. The usefulness of a symbolic approach to the cross-cultural study of attachment here becomes apparent. The interactional routines that give rise to individual differences in attachment behavior are affected not only by parental idiosyncrasies, but also by the cultural meaning systems that serve to shape parental perceptions, expectations, goals, values, discourse, and behaviors in culturally meaningful ways.

For example, Anglo mothers in our studies placed a great deal of emphasis on a child's Self-Maximization as an autonomous unit. They wanted their children to grow up to be self-confident, independent, happy, and able to fulfill their inner talents and potential. Concomitantly, they found the active A1 and B1 toddlers to be significantly more desirable than did the Puerto Rican mothers, and described what they liked and didn't like about all the toddlers in terms of the presence or absence of these self-maximizing qualities. Their perceptions thus reflected the individualism of dominant U.S. culture.

However, Anglo mothers also seemed to be acutely aware that an excess of individualism can be as problematic as its absence. Accordingly, they expressed the belief that a balance between Self-Maximization and the ability to relate to others was optimal, and their perceptions of the hypothetical toddlers reflected these concerns. The A1 toddler was liked for independence but criticized for emotional detachment, whereas the B4 toddler was praised for emotional connectedness to the mother but disliked for clinginess; the other Group B toddlers were considered to possess a healthy balance of independence and relatedness. A concern for control of negative emotions also emerged, with the ability to appropriately express and modulate tendencies toward aggression, selfishness, and egotism considered a further index of Self-Maximization; the C1 toddler was criticized for a lack of control over these negative emotional tendencies.

The Puerto Rican mothers, on the other hand, emphasized the importance of Proper Demeanor in interpersonal relationships. A child who demonstrates Proper Demeanor is respectful, calm, courteous, attentive to others, and able to gauge the level of behavioral decorum required by different social contexts. However, the Puerto Rican mothers were also concerned that their children possess the capacity for warmth, affection, and trust or intimacy, as well as the ability to know which level of relatedness is appropriate in which context. The Puerto Rican mothers thus liked the B2 and B3 toddlers for their ability to combine a calm, respectful demeanor with warmth and affection; they criticized the active A1 and B1 toddlers, as well as the C1 toddler, for their lack of proper demeanor. Although they appreciated the B4 toddler's closeness to the mother, they were concerned that this child would "suffer too much" when left alone.

The Puerto Rican mothers thus conceptualized desirable and undesirable toddler behaviors in a way that does not map directly onto the autonomy–relatedness dimension used by U.S. researchers to conceptualize the Strange Situation continuum. Instead, they appeared concerned that their children show a balance between a calm activity level and a positive engagement with the environment. Optimal balances for both cultures were more likely to fall in the middle (Group B) range of the continuum than at either of its ends; however, the continuum itself appeared to be defined differently across the two groups. Whereas the Anglo mothers conceptualized desirable and undesirable Strange Situation behavior, as well as the primary tasks of socialization, in terms of an optimal balance between autonomy and relatedness, the Puerto Rican mothers appeared to think in terms of a balance between Proper Demeanor and positive engagement. It is possible that for the Puerto Rican mothers, quiet but passively nonengaged children would be placed at one end of this continuum, while noisy, disruptive, angry children would be grouped together at the other end.

These studies examined only parental meaning systems, and so nothing can be concluded regarding parental antecedents to individual differences in attachment behavior among Puerto Rican versus Anglo mothers. However, on the basis of the existing literature, we would anticipate that warm, consistent parenting would predict Group B attachment outcomes in both groups. For both Anglo and Puerto Rican mothers, parental warmth and consistency would convey the sense of psychological safety that Bowlby and Ainsworth hypothesized to be essential to the development of Group B patterns of attachment. On the other hand, the concept of "security," although technically similar to a sense of psychological safety, has become laden with an array of values and ideals peculiar to mainstream U.S. discourse: The "secure" person is self-confident, independent, and able to utilize his or her talents and abilities to the fullest, but also has the capacity to be empathic and to relate to others. In short, the "secure" individual is one who embodies U.S. ideals of optimal socioemotional develop-ment—ideals that may or may not translate well into the meaning systems of other cultural groups.

These studies thus highlight the need for investigators to take cultural meaning systems into account when attempting to understand individual differences in attachment behavior. Such an approach may enhance the predictive power of individual differences in attachment in cultures outside of the United States by embedding those behaviors within culturally relevant symbolic frameworks. We may indeed find that Group B infants across many cultures perform well on tests of socioemotional development designed with dominant U.S. constructs in mind; for instance, we may find that prechoolers with Group B attachment history are more ego-resilient in Japan, Germany, and Israel, as well as in the United States. However, this leaves unanswered the relationship between Group B attachment and more culturally specific socialization goals. Embedding cross-cultural attachment re-search in indigenous meaning systems may serve to enhance the paradigm's usefulness in culturally diverse settings.

A symbolic approach to the study of desirable and undesirable child behavior may be particularly valuable when investigators are considering ethnic minorities within the United States, such as the working-class Puerto Rican mothers sampled in the present research. As has been described, these mothers are likely to hold cultural be-liefs and values concerning child rearing that differ markedly from those of the Anglo culture. At the same time, they are also likely to be considered "high-risk" mothers because of a variety of factors that tend to co-occur in this population, including poverty, unemployment, single-parent status, young maternal age, and school dropout status (Amaro & Russo, 1987). It is therefore important that researchers come to understand culturally sensitive norms regarding what being a "good child" or a "good parent" means for this sociocultural group.

Laosa (1979) speaks to this issue when he notes that a child "is perceived as socially competent or incompetent in the context of spe-cific roles and value judgments. The dominant group, however, has determined the characteristics that define a competent child" (p. 265). This is problematic when "someone unfamiliar with . . . the child's minority socioculture has defined (a) the context or situation in which performance is assessed and (b) the content and form of the tasks employed to assess competence" (p. 265). In this situation, one might "mistakenly equate cultural characteristics with deficiencies or mistakenly define as a deficiency a characteristic that may actually represent a cultural difference" (p. 270). The challenge for those who study and work with parents and children from sociocultural backgrounds different from their own is thus twofold. Theoretically, it is necessary to understand socially competent behavior as it is conceived by the sociocultural group in question, in order not to "mistakenly equate cultural characteristics with deficiencies"; practically, any sound intervention program must be sensitive to and able to educate all concerned regarding normative standards in the diverse contexts (both the dominant and the minority culture) in which these children will be required to function (Harwood & Weissberg, 1992).

In terms of socioeconomic status, the present results suggest that social class differences in perceptions of child behavior must be considered within the larger context of cultural values. In particular, although the working-class Anglo mothers endorsed dominant U.S. values regarding Self-Maximization, they seemed to view its attainment as potentially problematic, and concomitantly also emphasized other qualities, such as Decency and Proper Demeanor. In contrast, the working-class Puerto Rican mothers focused almost exclusively on culturally valued qualities falling within the domain of Proper Demeanor, while their middle-class counterparts tempered an emphasis on Proper Demeanor with attention to behavior falling within other categories as well. Thus, the working-class Anglo mothers seemed to steel themselves against a partial failure to attain culturally desired qualities, whereas working-class Puerto Rican mothers embraced culturally prescribed qualities with almost single-minded devotion. It would seem, then, that larger cultural values take on more specific, localized meanings among different social groups.

Finally, attachment behavior appears to provide a very rich vantage point from which to examine cultural meaning systems. As noted earlier, we can learn a great deal about the interpretation and negotiation of everyday social interactions from whether a toddler's active play is interpreted positively or negatively by caretakers, according to cultural constructs that place maximal value on Self-Maximization or Proper Demeanor.

An examination of normative development in the context of indigenous meaning systems can also enrich our understanding of what constitute ideal endpoints for socioemotional development. The emphasis in dominant U.S. culture on the development of the self as an autonomous unit may produce assertive adults who can maximize their chances for success and happiness in a mobile and competitive society. However, as several researchers have noted, this excessive individualism can also lead to alienation, narcissism, and spiritual emptiness (see Bellah et al., 1985; Cushman, 1990, 1991; Lasch, 1978; Sampson, 1989). As diagnoses of classical neuroses decrease while disorders of the self appear to increase, we as psychologists have a responsibility to engage in reflective self-criticism of the ideal endpoints that we endorse (Marcus & Fischer, 1986; Wartofsky, 1986). On the other hand, too much emphasis on traditional cultural values, such as *obediencia* and *respeto* in Puerto Rico, may hinder the individual's potential to bring about beneficial changes at the societal level. A greater understanding of alternative models of normative development may help us gain a greater understanding of the culture-boundness of any vision of the Good, as well as supply us with other ways of conceptualizing socioemotional endpoints.

Vignettes of Strange Situation Behavior Used in Study 2

♦

The gender of each toddler in the vignettes that follow was varied according to the gender of each mother's Strange Situation-age child. Note that the English names used are gender-neutral. (As noted in Chapter Five, each toddler was given a gender-appropriate Puerto Rican name in the Spanish translations of the vignettes; however, the English names are used throughout this book for the sake of simplicity.)

A1 TODDLER

This story is about Alex. Alex comes into the waiting room with her mother. Her mother sits on the couch. Alex looks around the room and notices the toys. "Would you like a toy?" her mother says as Alex walks over to where the toys are. Alex picks up a ball and begins bouncing it against the floor. After a minute, she tosses the ball toward the middle of the room. She then picks up another toy and walks over to the empty chair. She sets the toy on the seat of the chair and begins running it along the seat and side of the chair, as though it is a car she is pushing along. She makes humming sounds as she does this.

After another minute, the receptionist says to the mother that the doctor will see her now, and says she'll keep an eye on Alex for the few minutes that the mother will be gone. The mother says to Alex, "I'll be right back," and leaves the room. Alex does not look up from what she is doing. After her mother is gone, Alex moves the toy she is playing with to the floor and begins pushing it around the room. Then she goes back to the chair and climbs on it, standing there and shaking the toy she is holding. Then she gets down and picks up another toy. She examines it and then hits it against the chair.

After a few minutes, her mother returns to the waiting room and says, "Hi, Alex." Alex does not look up from what she is doing. While her mother is setting up another appointment, Alex wanders over to the front door, trying to reach the doorknob, until her mother is ready to leave the office.

BI TODDLER

This story is about Lee. Lee comes into the waiting room with his mother. His mother sits on the couch. Lee looks around the room and notices the toys. "Would you like a toy?" his mother says as Lee walks over to where the toys are. He picks up a ball and bounces it on the floor. He shows the ball to his mother, smiling and vocalizing. He then picks up another toy and begins pushing it around on the floor near the empty chair, as though it is a car he is pushing along. He makes humming sounds as he does this. He shows the toy to his mother again, smiling and vocalizing.

After another minute, the receptionist says to the mother that the doctor will see her now, and says she'll keep an eye on Lee for the few minutes that the mother will be gone. The mother says to Lee, "I'll be right back," and leaves the room. Lee looks up from his play. He pauses as he watches his mother leave. After a few seconds he selects another toy and continues playing, making humming sounds.

After a few minutes, his mother returns to the waiting room and says, "Hi, Lee." Lee looks up. He smiles and vocalizes happily, showing his mother the toy he has. He continues with his play until they are ready to leave the office a few minutes later.

B2 TODDLER

This story is about Kelly. Kelly comes into the waiting room with her mother. Her mother sits on the couch. She says to Kelly, "Would you like a toy?" Kelly walks over to the toys, and picks one up. She shows it to her mother, smiling and vocalizing. She sits down and begins to play with it. She pushes it around on the floor as though it's a car she is pushing along. She makes humming sounds as she does this. After a minute, she looks up at her mother and smiles, showing her the toy. She gets up, gets another toy, and begins playing with it.

After another minute, the receptionist says to the mother that the doctor will see her now, and says she'll keep an eye on Kelly for a few minutes that the mother will be gone. The mother says to Kelly, "I'll be right back," and leaves the room. Kelly follows her mother to the door and watches her leave the room. After a few seconds she returns to play. She looks up now and then at the door her mother disappeared through.

After a few minutes, her mother returns to the waiting room and says, "Hi, Kelly." Kelly gets up and comes over to her mother to be picked up, smiling and vocalizing happily. Her mother holds her for several seconds while she sets up another appointment, then puts her down. After a minute the mother is ready to leave, and they walk together out of the office.

B3 TODDLER

This story is about Pat. Pat comes into the waiting room with his mother. His mother sits on the couch. Pat sits next to his mother on the couch. After a minute, Pat's mother says to him, "Would you like a toy?" Pat looks at his mother, then at the toys. He gets up, gets a toy, and brings it back to the couch. He shows it to his mother, smiling and vocalizing. He then sits down next to his mother and plays quietly with the toy. Every once in a while he looks up at his mother.

After another minute, the receptionist says to the mother that the doctor will see her now, and says she'll keep an eye on Pat for the few minutes that the mother will be gone. The mother says to Pat, "I'll be right back," and leaves the room. Pat pauses as he watches his mother leave the room. He stays where he is on the couch, playing quietly with the toy.

After a few minutes, his mother returns to the waiting room and says, "Hi, Pat." Pat gets up and comes over to his mother, smiling and vocalizing. He reaches out his arms to be picked up. His mother holds him while she sets up another appointment. Pat hugs his mother closely and smiles. After a few minutes, Pat's mother puts him down. Pat reaches up to hold his mother's hand as they walk together out of the office.

B4 TODDLER

This story is about Chris. Chris comes into the waiting room with her mother. Her mother sits on the couch. Chris sits next to her mother on the couch. Chris's mother says to her, "Would you like a toy?" Chris looks at the toys, then at her mother. She reaches out her arms to be held. Chris's mother picks her up and holds her on her lap.

After another minute, the receptionist says to the mother that the doctor will see her now, and says she'll keep an eye on Chris for the few minutes that the mother will be gone. The mother says to Chris, "I'll be right back," and leaves the room. Chris gets up and follows her mother to the door. She begins crying as her mother leaves. The receptionist says, "It's okay, she'll be right back." Chris stays by the door. She cries and sucks her thumb while her mother is gone.

After a few minutes, her mother returns to the waiting room and says, "Hi, Chris." Chris, still crying, runs to her to be picked up. She clings tightly to her mother, still crying. After a minute, her mother tries to put her down, but she resists, still clinging. Chris's mother holds her until they are ready to leave the office.

C1 TODDLER

This story is about Lindsay. Lindsay comes into the waiting room with his mother. His mother sits on the couch. His mother says to him, "Would you like a toy?" Lindsay walks over, picks up several toys, and brings them back to the couch. He climbs onto his mother's lap with the toys. He whimpers, then throws the toy he is holding onto the floor.

After another minute, the receptionist says to the mother that the doctor will see her now, and says she'll keep an eye on Lindsay for the few minutes that the mother will be gone. The mother says to Lindsay, "I'll be right back," and leaves the room. Lindsay gets up and follows his mother to the door, beginning to cry. The receptionist says, "It's okay, she'll be right back." Lindsay stays by the door. He cries and sucks his thumb while his mother is gone.

After a few minutes, his mother returns to the waiting room and says, "Hi, Lindsay." Lindsay kicks and throws the toy he is holding onto the floor, still crying. His mother tries to pick him up, but Lindsay pushes away. He remains crying until they are ready to leave the office.

References

◆

Ainsworth, M. D. S. (1984) *Adaptation and attachment*. Paper presented at the International Conference on Infant Studies, New York.

Ainsworth, M. D. S., Bell, S. M., & Stayton, D. J. (1971). Individual differences in strange-situation behavior of one-year-olds. In H. R. Schaffer (Ed.), *The origins of human social relations* (pp. 17–57). London: Academic Press.

Ainsworth, M. D. S., Blehar, M. C., Waters, E., & Wall, S. (1978). *Patterns of attachment: A psychological study of the Strange Situation*. Hillsdale, NJ: Erlbaum.

Ainsworth, M. D. S., & Wittig, B. A. (1969). Attachment and exploratory behavior of one-year-olds in a strange situation. In B. M. Foss (Ed.), *Determinants of infant behavior* (pp. 111–136). London: Methuen.

Alexander, J. C., & Seidman, S. (Eds.). (1990). *Culture and society: Contemporary debates*. Cambridge, England: Cambridge University Press.

Amaro, H., & Russo, N. F. (1987). Hispanic women and mental health: An overview of contemporary issues in research and practice. *Psychology of Women Quarterly, 11*, 393–407.

Arend, R., Gove, F. L., & Sroufe, L. A. (1979). Continuity of individual adaptation from infancy to kindergarten: A predictive study of ego-resiliency and curiosity in preschoolers. *Child Development, 50*, 950–959.

Austin, J. L. (1975). *How to do things with words* (2nd ed). Cambridge, MA: Harvard University Press.

Barker, R. G., & Gump, P. V. (1964). *Big school, small school: High school size and student behavior*. Stanford, CA: Stanford University Press.

Barry, H., Child, I. L., & Bacon, M. K. (1959). Relation of child training to subsistence economy. *American Anthropologist, 61*, 51–63.

Bellah, R. N., Madsen, R., Sullivan, W. M., Swidler, A., & Tipton, S. M. (1985). *Habits of the heart: Individualism and commitment in American life*. Berkeley: University of California Press.

Belsky, J., & Nezworski, T. (Eds.). (1988). *Clinical implications of attachment*. Hillsdale, NJ: Erlbaum.

Benedict, R. (1934). *Patterns of culture*. Boston: Houghton Mifflin.

Berger, P. L., & Luckmann, T. (1966). *The social construction of reality: A treatise in the sociology of knowledge*. Garden City, NY: Doubleday.

Bethell, L. (Ed.). (1986). *The Cambridge history of Latin America: vol. 5. c. 1870 to 1930*. Cambridge, England: Cambridge University Press.

Bethell, L. (Ed.). (1990). *The Cambridge history of Latin America: Vol. 7. Latin America since 1930: Mexico, Central America and the Caribbean*. Cambridge, England: Cambridge University Press.

Blumer, H. (1987). Symbolic interaction. In J. P. Spradley (Ed.), *Culture and cognition: Rules, maps, and plans* (pp. 65–83). Prospect Heights, IL: Waveland Press.

Blumer, H. (1990). In D. R. Maines & T. J. Morrione (Eds.), *Industrialization as an agent of social change: A critical analysis*. New York: Aldine de Gruyter.

Bourdieu, P. (1991). *Language and symbolic power*. Cambridge, MA: Harvard University Press.

Bowlby, J. (1969). *Attachment and loss: Vol. 1. Attachment*. New York: Basic Books.

Bowlby, J. (1973). *Attachment and loss: Vol. 2. Separation: Anxiety and anger*. New York: Basic Books.

Bowlby, J. (1980). *Attachment and loss: Vol. 3. Loss: Sadness and depression*. New York: Basic Books.

Boyd, R., & Richerson, P. J. (1985). *Culture and the evolutionary process*. Chicago: University of Chicago Press.

Bretherton, I. (1985). Attachment theory: Retrospect and prospect. In I. Bretherton & E. Waters (Eds.), Growing points of attachment theory and research. *Monographs of the Society for Research in Child Development, 50*(1–2, Serial No. 209), 3–35.

Bretherton, I., & Waters, E. (Eds.). (1985). Growing points of attachment theory and research. *Monographs of the Society for Research in Child Development, 50* (1–2, Serial No. 209).

Briggs, C. L. (1986). *Learning how to ask: A sociolinguistic appraisal of the role of the interview in social science research*. Cambridge, England: Cambridge University Press.

Briggs, J. L. (1970). *Never in anger: Portrait of an Eskimo family*. Cambridge, MA: Harvard University Press.

Bronfenbrenner, U. (1977). Toward an experimental ecology of human development. *American Psychologist, 32*, 513–531.

Bruner, J. (1986). Value presuppositions of developmental theory. In L. Cirillo & S. Wapner (Eds.), *Value presuppositions in theories of human development* (pp. 19–28). Hillsdale, NJ: Erlbaum.

Bruner, J. (1990). *Acts of meaning*. Cambridge, MA: Harvard University Press.

Cahan, E. D. (1992). John Dewey and human development. *Developmental Psychology, 28*, 205–214.

Cahan, E. D., & White, S. H. (1992). Proposals for a second psychology. *American Psychologist, 47*, 224–235.

Carr, R. (1984). *Puerto Rico: A colonial experiment*. New York: Vintage.

Centro de Estudios Puertorriqueños. (1979). *Labor migration under capitalism: The Puerto Rican experience*. New York: Monthly Review Press.

Clifford, J. (1986). Partial truths. In J. Clifford & G. E. Marcus (Eds.), *Writing culture: The poetics and politics of ethnography* (pp. 1–26). Berkeley: University of California Press.

Cohen, R. (1978). Ethnicity: Problem and focus in anthropology. *Annual Review of Anthropology, 7*, 379–403.

Cole, M. (1983). Society, mind, and development. In F. S. Kessel & A. W. Siegel (Eds.), *The child and other cultural inventions* (pp. 89–114). New York: Praeger.

Cole, M. (1985). The zone of proximal development: Where culture and cognition create each other. In J. V. Wertsch (Ed.), *Culture, communication, and cognition: Vygotskian perspectives* (pp. 146–161). Cambridge, England: Cambridge University Press.

Corsaro, W. A., & Miller, P. J. (Eds.). (1992). Interpretive approaches to children's socialization. *New Directions for Child Development, 58*.

Crespo, E. (1986). A regional variation: Emotions in Spain. In R. Harre (Ed.), *The social construction of emotions* (pp. 209–217). Oxford: Blackwell.

Cushman, P. (1990). Why the self is empty: Toward a historically situated psychology. *American Psychologist, 45*, 599–611.

Cushman, P. (1991). Ideology obscured: Political uses of the self in Daniel Stern's infant. *American Psychologist, 46*, 206–219.

D'Andrade, R. (1992). Schemas and motivation. In R. D'Andrade & C. Strauss (Eds.), *Human motives and cultural models* (pp. 23–44). Cambridge, England: Cambridge University Press.

D'Andrade, R., & Strauss, C. (Eds.). (1992). *Human motives and cultural models*. Cambridge, England: Cambridge University Press.

Denzin, N., & Lincoln, Y. (1994). *Handbook of qualitative research*. Thousand Oaks, CA: Sage.

Derrida, J. (1978). *Writing and difference*. London: Routledge.

deVries, M. W. (1984). Temperament and infant mortality among the Masai of East Africa. *American Journal of Psychiatry, 141*, 1189–1194.

Diaz Royo, A. (1974). *The enculturation process of Puerto Rican highland children* (Doctoral dissertation, University of Michigan). (University Microfilms No. 75-12506,324).

Dilthey, W. (1985). *Selected works: Vol. 1. Introduction to the human sciences* (R. A. Makkreel & F. Rodi, Eds. and Trans.). Princeton, NJ: Princeton University Press. (Original work published 1883–1893)

Dixon, S., Tronick, E., Keefer, C., & Brazelton, T. B. (1981). Mother–infant interaction among the Gusii of Kenya. In T. Field, A. Sostek, P. Vietze,

& P. Leiderman (Eds.), *Culture and early interaction* (pp. 149–168). Hillsdale, NJ: Erlbaum.

Drummond, L. (1980). The cultural continuum: A theory of intersystems. *Man, 15,* 352–374.

Dumont, L. (1986). *Essays on individualism: Modern ideology in anthropological perspective.* Chicago: University of Chicago Press.

Dunn, J. (1987). The beginnings of moral understanding: Development in the second year. In J. Kagan & S. Lamb (Eds.), *The emergence of morality in young children* (pp. 91–122). Chicago: University of Chicago Press.

Dworkin, G. (1988). *The theory and practice of autonomy.* Cambridge, England: Cambridge University Press.

Ermarth, M. (1978). *Wilhelm Dilthey: The critique of historical reason.* Chicago: University of Chicago Press.

Fiske, D. W., & Shweder, R. A. (Eds.). (1986). *Metatheory in social science: Pluralisms and subjectivities.* Chicago: University of Chicago Press.

Gadamer, H. G. (1975). *Truth and method.* New York: Seabury.

Garbarino, J. (1990). The human ecology of early risk. In S. Meisels & J. Shonkoff (Eds.), *Handbook of early childhood intervention* (pp. 78–96). Cambridge, England: Cambridge University Press.

Garfinkel, H. (1967). *Studies in ethnomethodology.* Englewood Cliffs, NJ: Prentice-Hall.

Garvey, C. (Ed.). (1992). Talk in the study of socialization and development [Special issue]. *Merrill–Palmer Quarterly, 38.*

Gecas, V. (1979). The influence of social class on socialization. In W. R. Burr, R. Hill, F. I. Nye, & I. L. Reiss (Eds.), *Contemporary theories about the family* (pp. 365–404). New York: Free Press.

Geertz, C. (1973). *The interpretation of cultures.* New York: Basic Books.

Geertz, C. (1984). "From the native's point of view": On the nature of anthropological understanding. In R. A. Shweder & R. A. LeVine (Eds.), *Culture theory: Essays on mind, self, and emotion* (pp. 124–136). Cambridge, England: Cambridge University Press.

Gergen, K. J. (1985). The social constructionist movement in modern psychology. *American Psychologist, 40,* 266–275.

Gewirtz, J. L., & Kurtines, W. M. (Eds.). (1991). *Intersections with attachment.* Hillsdale, NJ: Erlbaum.

Giddens, A. (1973). *The class structure of the advanced societies.* London: Hutchinson University Library.

Giddens, A. (1976). *New rules of sociological method: A positive critique of interpretative sociologies.* New York: Basic Books.

Giddens, A. (1987). *Social theory and modern sociology.* Stanford, CA: Stanford University Press.

Gollin, E., Stahl, G., & Morgan, E. (1989). On the uses of the concept of normality in developmental biology and psychology. In H. W. Reese

(Ed.), *Advances in child development and behavior* (pp. 49–71). New York: Academic Press.

Gould, S. J. (1980). *The panda's thumb: More reflections in natural history.* New York: Norton.

Gould, S. J., & Lewontin, R. C. (1979). The spandrels of San Marco and the Panglossian paradigm: A critique of the adaptationist programme. *Proceedings of the Royal Society of London, B205,* 581–598.

Grossmann, K., Grossmann, K. E., Spangler, G., Suess, G., & Unzner, L. (1985). Maternal sensitivity and newborns' orientation responses as related to quality of attachment in northern Germany. In I. Bretherton & E. Waters (Eds.), Growing points of attachment theory and research. *Monographs of the Society for Research in Child Development, 50* (1–2, Serial No. 209), 233–256.

Grossmann, K. E., & Grossmann, K. (1990). The wider concept of attachment in cross-cultural research. *Human Development, 33,* 31–47.

Gumperz, J. J. (1972). The speech community. In P. P. Giglioli (Ed.), *Language and social context* (pp. 219–231). Harmondsworth, England: Penguin Books.

Gumperz, J. J. (1982). *Discourse strategies.* Cambridge, England: Cambridge University Press.

Gumperz, J. J., & Hymes, D. (Eds.). (1986). *Directions in sociolinguistics: The ethnography of communication.* Oxford: Blackwell.

Gunnar, M. R., & Sroufe, L. A. (Eds.). (1991). *Self processes and development.* Hillsdale, NJ: Erlbaum.

Harkness, S., & Super, C. M. (1985). Child–environment interactions in the socialization of affect. In M. Lewis & C. Saarni (Eds.), *The socialization of emotions* (pp. 21–36). New York: Plenum.

Harkness, S., & Super, C. M. (1992). Parental ethnotheories in action. In I. E. Sigel, A. V. McGillicuddy-DeLisi, & J. J. Goodnow (Eds.), *Parental belief systems: The psychological consequences for children* (2nd ed., pp. 373–391). Hillsdale, NJ: Erlbaum.

Harkness, S., Super, C. M., & Keefer, C. H. (1992). Learning to be an American parent: How cultural models gain directive force. In R. D'Andrade & C. Strauss (Eds.), *Human motives and cultural models* (pp. 163–178). Cambridge, England: Cambridge University Press.

Harwood, R. L. (1992). The influence of culturally derived values on Anglo and Puerto Rican mothers' perceptions of attachment behavior. *Child Development, 63,* 822–839.

Harwood, R. L., & Miller, J. G. (1991). Perceptions of attachment behavior: A comparison of Anglo and Puerto Rican mothers. *Merrill–Palmer Quarterly, 37,* 583–599.

Harwood, R. L., Ventura-Cook, E., Schulze, P. A., & Wilson, S. P. (1995). *Anglo and Puerto Rican mothers' beliefs regarding long-term socialization goals and child behavior: Culture, class, and sociodemographic characteristics as multiple ecological sources.* Manuscript submitted for publication.

Harwood, R. L., & Weissberg, R. P. (1992). A conceptual framework for context-sensitive prevention programming: A symbolic interactionist perspective. *Journal of Primary Prevention, 13*, 85–113.

Heath, S. B. (1986). What no bedtime story means: Narrative skills at home and school. In B. Schieffelin & E. Ochs (Eds.), *Language socialization across cultures* (pp. 97–124). Cambridge, England: Cambridge University Press.

Hess, R. D. (1970). Social class and ethnic influences upon socialization. In P. H. Mussen (Ed.), *Carmichael's manual of child psychology* (3rd ed., pp. 457–557). New York: Wiley.

Hinde, R. A. (1982). Attachment: Some conceptual and biological issues. In C. M. Parkes & J. Stevenson-Hinde (Eds.), *The place of attachment in human behavior* (pp. 60–76). London: Tavistock.

Hinde, R. A., & Stevenson-Hinde, J. (1990). Attachment: Biological, cultural and individual desiderata. *Human Development, 33*, 62–72.

Hoff-Ginsberg, E., & Tardif, T. (1995). Socioeconomic status and parenting. In M. H. Bornstein (Ed.), *Handbook of parenting*. Hillsdale, NJ: Erlbaum.

Hollingshead, A. B. (1975). *Four factor index of social status*. Unpublished manuscript, Yale University.

Howard, G. S. (1985). The role of values in the science of psychology. *American Psychologist, 40*, 255–265.

Hsu, F. L. K. (Ed.). (1961). *Psychological anthropology: Approaches to culture and personality*. Homewood, IL: Dorsey Press.

Husserl, E. (1960). *Cartesian meditations: An introduction to phenomenology*. The Hague: Martinus Nijhoff.

Jackman, M. R., & Jackman, R. W. (1983). *Class awareness in the United States*. Berkeley: University of California Press.

Keesing, R. M. (1981). Theories of culture. In R. W. Casson (Ed.), *Language, culture, and cognition: Anthropological perspectives* (pp. 42–66). New York: Macmillan.

Kessen, W. (Ed.). (1965). *The child*. New York: Wiley.

Kessen, W. (1979). The American child and other cultural inventions. *American Psychologist, 34*, 815–820.

Kohn, M. L. (1977). *Class and conformity: A study in values* (2nd ed.). Chicago: University of Chicago Press.

Laboratory of Comparative Human Cognition. (1983). Culture and cognitive development. In W. Kessen (Vol. Ed.), *Handbook of child psychology* (4th ed.): *Vol. 1. History, theory, and methods* (pp. 295–356). New York: Wiley.

LaFreniere, P. J., & Sroufe, L. A. (1985). Profiles of peer competence in the preschool: Interrelations between measures, influence of social ecology, and relation to attachment history. *Child Development, 21*, 56–69.

Lakoff, G., & Johnson, M. (1980). *Metaphors we live by*. Chicago: University of Chicago Press.

Lamb, M. E., Thompson, R. A., Gardner, W., & Charnov, E. L. (1985). *Infant–mother attachment: The origins and developmental significance of individual differences in Strange Situation behavior*. Hillsdale, NJ: Erlbaum.

Laosa, L. M. (1979). Social competence in childhood: Toward a developmental, socioculturally relativistic paradigm. In M. W. Kent & J. E. Rolf (Eds.), *Primary prevention of psychopathology* (pp. 253–279). Hanover, NH: University Press of New England.

Lasch, C. (1978). *The culture of narcissism: American life in an age of diminishing expectations*. New York: Norton.

Lauria, A. (1982). *Respeto, relajo*, and interpersonal relations in Puerto Rico. In F. Cordasco & E. Bucchioni (Eds.), *The Puerto Rican community and its children on the mainland* (2nd ed., pp. 58–71). Metuchen, NJ: Scarecrow Press.

LeVine, R. A. (1973). *Culture, behavior, and personality*. Chicago: Aldine.

Levy, R. (1980). *On the nature and functions of the emotions: An anthropological perspective*. Unpublished manuscript.

Lewis, M. (1989). What do we mean when we say emotional development? In L. Cirillo, B. Kaplan, & S. Wapner (Eds.), *Emotions in ideal human development* (pp. 53–75). Hillsdale, NJ: Erlbaum.

Lewis, M., & Saarni, C. (Eds.). (1985). *The socialization of emotions*. New York: Plenum.

Little, D. (1991). *Varieties of social explanation: An introduction to the philosophy of social science*. Boulder, CO: Westview Press.

Londerville, S., & Main, M. (1981). Security of attachment, compliance, and maternal training methods in the second year of life. *Developmental Psychology, 17*, 289–299.

Lovejoy, A. O. (1936). *The great chain of being*. Cambridge, MA: Harvard University Press.

Lucca, N. (1988). Self-understanding in a Puerto Rican fishing village. In W. Damon & D. Hart (Eds.), *Self-understanding in childhood and adolescence* (pp. 158–198). Cambridge, England: Cambridge University Press.

Lutz, C. A. (1990). Engendered emotion: Gender, power, and the rhetoric of emotional control in American discourse. In C. Lutz & L. Abu-Lughod (Eds.), *Language and the politics of emotions* (pp. 69–92). Cambridge, England: Cambridge University Press.

Lutz, C. A., & White, G. M. (1986). The anthropology of emotions. *Annual Review of Anthropology, 15*, 405–436.

Main, M., Kaplan, N., & Cassidy, J. (1985). Security in infancy, childhood, and adulthood: A move to the level of representation. In I. Bretherton

& E. Waters (Eds.), Growing points of attachment theory and research. *Monographs of the Society for Research in Child Development, 50* (1–2, Serial No. 209), 66–104.

Main, M., & Solomon, J. (1986). Discovery of an insecure–disorganized/disoriented attachment pattern. In T. B. Brazelton & M. W. Yogman (Eds.), *Affective development in infancy* (pp. 95–124). Norwood, NJ: Ablex.

Main, M., & Weston, D. R. (1982). Avoidance of the attachment figure in infancy: Descriptions and interpretations. In C. M. Parkes & J. Stevenson-Hinde (Eds.), *The place of attachment in human behavior* (pp. 31– 59). London: Tavistock.

Malatesta, C., & Haviland, J. (1985). The modification of emotional expression in human development. In M. Lewis & C. Saarni (Eds.), *The socialization of emotions* (pp. 89–116). New York: Plenum.

Malinowski, B. (1927). *Sex and repression in savage society.* London: Routledge & Kegan Paul.

Mandelbaum, M. (1971). *History, man, and reason: A study in nineteenth-century thought.* Baltimore: Johns Hopkins University Press.

Manganaro, M. (Ed.). (1990). *Modernist anthropology: From fieldwork to text.* Princeton, NJ: Princeton University Press.

Marcus, G. E., & Fischer, M. M. J. (1986). *Anthropology as cultural critique: An experimental moment in the human sciences.* Chicago: University of Chicago Press.

Marin, G., & Triandis, H. C. (1985). Allocentrism as an important characteristic of the behavior of Latin Americans and Hispanics. In R. Diaz Guerrero (Ed.), *Cross-cultural and national studies in social psychology* (pp. 85–104). Amsterdam: Elsevier/North-Holland.

Markus, H. R., & Kitayama, S. (1991). Culture and the self: Implications for cognition, emotion, and motivation. *Psychological Review, 98,* 224–253.

Matas, L., Arend, R. A., & Sroufe, L. A. (1978). Continuity of adaptation in the second year: The relationship between quality of attachment and later competence. *Child Development, 49,* 547–556.

Mead, G. H. (1934). *Mind, self and society.* Chicago: University of Chicago Press.

Mead, M. (1928). *Coming of age in Samoa.* New York: Morrow.

Miller, J. G. (1984). Culture and the development of everyday social explanation. *Journal of Personality and Social Psychology, 46,* 961–978.

Miller, J. G. (1994). Cultural psychology: Bridging disciplinary boundaries in understanding the cultural grounding of self. In P. Bock (Ed.), *Handbook of psychological anthropology.* Westport, CT: Greenwood.

Miller, J. G., & Bersoff, D. M. (1992). Culture and moral judgment: How are conflicts between justice and interpersonal responsibilities resolved? *Journal of Personality and Social Psychology, 62,* 541–554.

Miller, J. G., Bersoff, D. M., & Harwood, R. L. (1990). Perceptions of social responsibilities in India and in the United States: Moral imperatives or personal decisions? *Journal of Personality and Social Psychology, 58*, 33–47.

Miller, P. J. (1982). *Amy, Wendy, and Beth: Learning language in South Baltimore*. Austin: University of Texas Press.

Miller, P. J., Mintz, J., Hoogstra, L., Fung, H., & Potts, R. (1992). The narrated self: Young children's construction of self in relation to others in conversational stories of personal experience. *Merrill–Palmer Quarterly, 38*, 45–67.

Miyake, K., Chen, S. J., & Campos, J. J. (1985). Infant temperament, mother's mode of interaction, and attachment in Japan: An interim report. In I. Bretherton & E. Waters (Eds.), Growing points of attachment theory and research. *Monographs of the Society for Research in Child Development, 50* (1–2, Serial No. 209), 276–297.

Morss, J. R. (1990). *The biologising of childhood: Developmental psychology and the Darwinian myth*. Hillsdale, NJ: Erlbaum.

Nakagawa, M., Lamb, M. E., & Miyake, K. (1988). Psychological experiences of Japanese infants in the Strange Situation. In *Research and Clinical Center for Child Development, Annual Report* (No. 11, pp. 13–24). Sapporo, Japan: Hokkaido University.

Ochs, E., & Schieffelin, B. B. (1984). Language acquisition and socialization: Three developmental stories and their implications. In R. A. Shweder & R. A. LeVine (Eds.), *Culture theory: Essays on mind, self, and emotion* (pp. 276–320). Cambridge, England: Cambridge University Press.

Odum, E. (1953). *Fundamentals of ecology*. Philadelphia: W. B. Saunders.

Ogbu, J. U. (1981). Origins of human competence: A cultural-ecological perspective. *Child Development, 52*, 413–429.

Oppenheim, D., Sagi, A., & Lamb, M. E. (1988). Infant–adult attachments on the kibbutz and their relation to socioemotional development 4 years later. *Developmental Psychology, 24*, 427–433.

Orlove, B. S. (1980). Ecological anthropology. *Annual Review of Anthropology, 9*, 235–269.

Parkes, C. M., & Stevenson-Hinde, J. (Eds.). (1982). *The place of attachment in human behavior*. London: Tavistock.

Perlmann, J. (1988). *Ethnic differences: Schooling and social structure among the Irish, Italians, Jews, and Blacks in an American city, 1880–1935*. Cambridge, England: Cambridge University Press.

Polanyi, L. (1989). *Telling the American story: A structural and cultural analysis of conversational storytelling*. Cambridge, MA: MIT Press.

Powers, M. G. (Ed.). (1982). *Measures of socioeconomic status: Current issues*. Boulder, CO: Westview Press.

Ricoeur, P. (1978). *The philosophy of Paul Ricoeur*. Boston: Beacon Press.

Roseberry, W. (1988). Political economy. *Annual Review of Anthropology, 17*, 161–185.

Roseberry, W. (1989). *Anthropologies and histories: Essays in culture, history, and political economy*. New Brunswick, NJ: Rutgers University Press.

Sagi, A. (1990). Attachment theory and research from a cross-cultural perspective. *Human Development, 33*, 10–22.

Sagi, A., van IJzendoorn, M.H., Aviezer, O., Donnell, F., & Mayseless, O. (1994). Sleeping out of home in a kibbutz communal arrangement: It makes a difference for infant–mother attachment. *Child Development, 65*, 992–1004.

Sagi, A., van IJzendoorn, M. H., & Koren-Karie, N. (1991). Primary appraisal of the Strange Situation: A cross-cultural analysis of preseparation episodes. *Developmental Psychology, 27*, 587–596.

Sahlins, M. (1976). *Culture and practical reason*. Chicago: University of Chicago Press.

Sampson, E. E. (1989). The challenge of social change for psychology: Globalization and psychology's theory of the person. *American Psychologist, 44*, 914–921.

Sargent, S. S., & Smith, M. W. (Eds.). (1949). *Culture and personality*. New York: Viking.

Saussure, F. (1974). *Course in general linguistics*. London: Fontana.

Scarr, S. (1985). Constructing psychology: Making facts and fables for our times. *American Psychologist, 40*, 499–512.

Scarr, S. (1992). Developmental theories for the 1990's: Developmental and individual differences. *Child Development, 63*, 1–19.

Schieffelin, B. B., & Ochs, E. (Eds.). (1986). *Language socialization across cultures*. Cambridge, England: Cambridge University Press.

Schneider, D. M., & Smith, R. T. (1978). *Class differences in American kinship*. Ann Arbor: University of Michigan Press.

Schutz, A. (1967). *The phenomenology of the social world*. Evanston, IL: Northwestern University Press.

Schwartz, B. (1990). The creation and destruction of value. *American Psychologist, 45*, 7–15.

Searle, J. (1972). What is a speech act? In P. P. Giglioli (Ed.), *Language and social context* (pp. 136–154). Harmondsworth, England: Penguin Books.

Segall, M. H., Dasen, P. R., Berry, J. W., & Poortinga, Y. H. (1990). *Human behavior in global perspective: An introduction to cross-cultural psychology*. Elmsford, NY: Pergamon Press.

Shweder, R. A. (1990). Cultural psychology—what is it? In J. W. Stigler, R. A. Shweder, & G. Herdt (Eds.), *Cultural psychology: Essays on comparative human development* (pp. 1–43). Cambridge, England: Cambridge University Press.

Shweder, R. A., & Bourne, E. J. (1984). Does the concept of the person vary cross-culturally? In R. A. Shweder & R. A. LeVine (Eds.), *Culture theory: Essays on mind, self, and emotion* (pp. 158–199). Cambridge, England: Cambridge University Press.

Sider, G. M. (1986). *Culture and class in anthropology and history: A New-foundland illustration.* Cambridge, England: Cambridge University Press.

Sigel, I. E., McGillicuddy-DeLisi, A. V., & Goodnow, J. J. (Eds.). (1992). *Parental belief systems: The psychological consequences for children* (2nd ed). Hillsdale, NJ: Erlbaum.

Smith, R. T. (1984). Anthropology and the concept of social class. *Annual Review of Anthropology, 13,* 467–494.

Spence, J. T. (1985). Achievement American style: The rewards and costs of individualism. *American Psychologist, 40,* 1285–1295.

Spencer, M. B., & Markstrom-Adams, C. (1990). Identity processes among racial and ethnic minority children in America. *Child Development, 61,* 290–310.

Spradley, J. P. (Ed.). (1972). *Culture and cognition: Rules, maps, and plans.* Prospect Heights, IL: Waveland Press.

Sroufe, L. A. (1988). The role of infant–caregiver attachment in development. In J. Belsky & T. Nesworski (Eds.), *Clinical implications of attachment* (pp. 18–38). Hillsdale, NJ: Erlbaum.

Sroufe, L. A., Egeland, B., & Kreutzer, T. (1990). The fate of early experience following developmental change: Longitudinal approaches to individual adaptation in childhood. *Child Development, 61,* 1363–1373.

Sroufe, L. A., Fox, N. E., & Pancake, V. R. (1983). Attachment and dependency in developmental perspective. *Child Development, 54,* 1615–1627.

Sroufe, L. A., & Waters, E. (1977). Attachment as an organizational construct. *Child Development, 48,* 1184–1199.

Stayton, D. J., & Ainsworth, M. D. S. (1973). Individual differences in infant responses to brief, everyday separations as related to other infant and maternal behaviors. *Developmental Psychology, 9,* 226–235.

Steward, J. H. (1955). *Theory of culture change: The methodology of multilinear evolution.* Urbana: University of Illinois Press.

Stocking, G. W. (Ed.). (1984). *Functionalism historicized: Essays on British social anthropology.* Madison: University of Wisconsin Press.

Strauss, C. (1992). What makes Tony run? Schemas as motives reconsidered. In R. D'Andrade & C. Strauss (Eds.), *Human motives and cultural models* (pp. 197–224). Cambridge, England: Cambridge University Press.

Super, C. M., & Harkness, S. (1986). The developmental niche: A conceptualization at the interface of child and culture. *International Journal of Behavioral Development, 9,* 545–569.

Takahashi, K. (1986). Examining the strange situation procedure with Japanese mothers and 12-month-old infants. *Developmental Psychology, 22,* 265–270.

Takahishi, K. (1990). Are the key assumptions of the "Strange Situation" procedure universal? A view from Japanese research. *Human Development, 33,* 23–30.

Tavecchio, L. W. C., & van IJzendoorn, M. H. (Eds.). (1987). *Attachment in social networks: Contributions to the Bowlby–Ainsworth attachment theory.* Amsterdam: Elsevier/North-Holland.

Tobin, J. J., Wu, D. Y. H., & Davidson, D. H. *Preschool in three cultures: Japan, China, and the United States.* New Haven, CT: Yale University Press.

Tomasello, M., Kruger, A. C., & Ratner, H. H. (1993). Cultural learning. *Behavioral and Brain Sciences, 16,* 495–552.

Tuan, Y. F. (1982). *Segmented worlds and self: Group life and individual consciousness.* Minneapolis: University of Minnesota Press.

Turiel, E. (1983). *The development of social knowledge: Morality and convention.* Cambridge, England: Cambridge University Press.

U.S. Bureau of the Census. (1990). *General population characteristics* (Series No. CP-1-8-53). Washington, DC: U.S. Government Printing Office.

van IJzendoorn, M. H. (Ed.). (1990). Cross-cultural validity of attachment theory [Special issue]. *Human Development, 33.*

van IJzendoorn, M. H., & Kroonenberg, P. M. (1988). Cross-cultural patterns of attachment: A meta-analysis of the Strange Situation. *Child Development, 59,* 147–156.

Vygotsky, L. S. (1978). *Mind in society: The development of higher psychological processes.* Cambridge, MA: Harvard University Press.

Wartofsky, M. W. (1983). The child's construction of the world and the world's construction of the child: From historical epistemology to historical psychology. In F. S. Kessel & A. W. Siegel (Ed.), *The child and other cultural inventions* (pp. 188–215). New York: Praeger.

Wartofsky, M. W. (1986). On the creation and transformation of norms of human development. In L. Cirillo & S. Wapner (Eds.), *Value presuppositions in theories of human development* (pp. 113–125). Hillsdale, NJ: Erlbaum.

Waters, E. (1978). The reliability and stability of individual differences in infant-mother attachment. *Child Development, 49,* 483–494.

Waters, E., Wippman, J., & Sroufe, L. A. (1979). Attachment, positive affect, and competence in the peer group: Two studies in construct validation. *Child Development, 50,* 821–829.

Wertsch, J. V. (1985). *Vygotsky and the social formation of mind.* Cambridge, MA: Harvard University Press.

White, L. A. (1959). *The evolution of culture: The development of civilization to the fall of Rome.* New York: McGraw-Hill.

White, S. (1983). The idea of development in developmental psychology. In R. M. Lerner (Ed.), *Developmental psychology: Historical and philosophical perspectives* (pp. 55–77). Hillsdale, NJ: Erlbaum.

Whiting, B. B., & Edwards, C. P. (1988). *Children of different worlds: The formation of social behavior.* Cambridge, MA: Harvard University Press.

Whiting, B. B., & Whiting, J. W. M. (1975). *Children of six cultures: A psychocultural analysis.* Cambridge, MA: Harvard University Press.

Whiting, J. W. M. (1961). Socialization processes and personality. In F. L. K. Hsu (Ed.), *Psychological anthropology: Approaches to culture and personality* (pp. 355–380). Homewood, IL: Dorsey Press.

Whiting, J. W. M. (1977). A model for psychocultural research. In P. Leiderman, S. Tulkin, & A. Rosenfeld (Eds.), *Culture and infancy* (pp. 29–47). New York: Academic Press.

Winch, P. (1958). *The idea of a social science and its relation to philosophy.* London: Routledge & Kegan Paul.

Wolf, E. R. (1982). *Europe and the people without history.* Berkeley: University of California Press.

Index

♦